What This Book Is About .

- This book shows you how to look into eyes and tell the body's inherent weaknesses and strengths.

- This book explains why some people are nearly always well in spite of their indiscretions, while others who try to take care of themselves are sick.

- This book explains the meaning of colors seen in the eyes and how eye color can be changed or modified.

- This book reveals what you can and cannot learn from the eyes using iridology.

- This book tells you the four most important things to take care of in order to gain and maintain better health.

- This book shows the importance of integrating other natural-health-care disciplines, especially nutrition, with iridology in order to build health.

Visions
of
Health

UNDERSTANDING IRIDIOLOGY

Dr. Bernard Jensen
Dr. Donald V. Bodeen

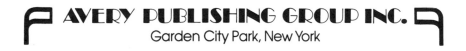
AVERY PUBLISHING GROUP INC.
Garden City Park, New York

The advice in this book is based on the personal experiences of the authors. Because each person and situation are unique, the editor and the publisher urge the reader to check with a qualified health professional when there is any question regarding the presence or treatment of any abnormal health condition. It is a sign of wisdom, not cowardice, to seek a second or third opinion.

The publisher does not advocate the use of any particular diet or treatment but believes the information presented in this book should be available to the public.

Cover design: Rudy Shur and Janine Eisner-Wall
Cover photo: Joyce Bodeen
In-house editor: Elaine Will Sparber
Typesetting: Coghill Book Typesetting Co., Richmond, VA

Library of Congress Cataloging-in-Publication Data

Jensen, Bernard.
    Visions of health / Bernard Jensen and Donald Bodeen.
      p.   cm.
    Includes bibliographical references and index.
    ISBN 0-89529-433-8
    1. Iridology. I. Bodeen, Donald. II. Title.
    [DNLM: 1. Eye Manifestations. 2. Iris. WW 475 J54v]
RC73.55.J47 1992
616.07'545—dc20
DNLM/DLC
for Library of Congress   91-21992
                                          CIP

Printed in the United States of America.
10 9 8 7 6 5 4 3 2

Contents

It sometimes seems a great sacrifice to dedicate one's life to a truth or a belief. Yet because of this unselfish application of certain individuals, truth takes on real meaning. I humbly acknowledge my gratitude to the mentors I have had who have, through their dedication, helped me to put light in dark places. I hope I have used their knowledge wisely for the benefit of the wholistic healing arts and mankind.

—B.J.

Iridology has been something of an orphan. No healing art in particular has seen fit to adopt it, to be identified with it. It is a fact of life that most new concepts are at first rebuffed. I have found iridology to be a most useful tool. Married to nutrition, it has been indispensable in practice. As with nutrition and all things ahead of their time, I believe, iridology's day in the sun is in the process of arriving.

—D.V.B.

Acknowledgments

The authors wish to thank their wives, Marie Jensen and Joyce Bodeen, without whose assistance and understanding, life would be infinitely more difficult.

We also wish to thank our publisher, the Avery Publishing Group, and its staff for all their kindness, patience, and professional assistance in the preparation of this book.

Foreword

Do you believe that you are what you eat? Today, the overwhelming majority of people will answer "yes." With this thought in mind, Dr. Bernard Jensen has dedicated his life to the search for good health through nutritional excellence. Internationally acclaimed and the author of numerous books, he has guided people to improve their quality of life and health by changing their eating habits. Dr. Jensen, at age 83—but looking twenty years younger!—is a living example of how we can achieve perfect harmony between the physical and the emotional. In addition, with improved nutritional habits, we can help to reduce the killer stress factor that is all too prevalent in our daily lives.

As a United Kingdom-trained chartered physiotherapist, I was attracted to iridology through my own medical and nutritional interests in association with my husband's profession as an optometrist. Fascinated by the wealth of information about the body that the eye reveals, I was drawn to the philosophies and ideals as expounded by Dr. Jensen in his books and seminars. It was at one of these seminars that I was fortunate enough to meet Dr. Donald Bodeen, whom, as Dr. Jensen's colleague, has contributed greatly towards the pioneering of iridology and its acceptance as an effective analytical method that can be used by all health practitioners.

The hope for the future is that the intensive research and analysis that are currently being undertaken will lead us to a greater understanding of our physical and nutritional needs to enable us to achieve a healthy and well-balanced lifestyle.

—Sheila Spivack, Grad. Dip. Phys., M.C.S.P., S.R.P.

Preface

I ridology is exciting! If you like excitement, you will like this book. The excitement of iridology stems from the thought that if tissue integrity throughout the body can be assessed by simply observing the color and structure of the iris, then a new and wonderful world of diagnostics and preventive medicine could thereby unfold before us. If this is so, why, you may ask, hasn't the science of iridology already made a smashing debut in the theatre of the healing arts? This book will tell you why. The science of iridology has been a sleeping giant. But of late, the giant has been stirring.

Iridology is controversial. Once you know what constitutes the science and practice of iris diagnosis, you will find it impossible to leave it alone. You will be compelled to investigate it in depth and then to either reject it or embrace it. You will find no middle ground. If iridology is true, it is nothing short of astounding, and the logical extensions of its philosophy will be enough to cause modern orthodox medicine to re-examine some of its most cherished principles. If false, it has to be the tragic product of misguided, albeit well-intentioned, people who mistakenly devoted the better part of their professional lives to its philosophy, practice, and promotion. But there is one thing iridology is not: it is not dull!

If you have eyes to see, iridology is for you. You don't have to be a health-care professional. You don't have to be a college graduate. And you don't have to be an expert to prove to yourself the validity and the benefits of reading the iris. The pages of this book will guide you step-by-step to the place where you, with no equipment other than a flashlight and simple magnifying glass, can examine your own eyes or the eyes of a friend and gain accurate and valuable information. How you utilize this information can be instrumental for you in attaining and maintaining health. You will learn how the eye is more than just "the window of the soul." Iridology will lend new meaning to the phrase, "the 'eyes' have it!" Let's not waste another moment. Enjoy!

Introduction

Iris analysis is catching on. It's coming out of seclusion. A technique once known and practiced by only a few, iridology—as it is called—is being discovered by a greater number of people. Founded in the late nineteenth century in Hungary, iris analysis is now being studied in many countries of the world. Not long ago, Soviet officials announced that it is being taught in medically oriented institutions in the U.S.S.R. The Chinese recently translated modern iridology textbooks into their language. Iris analysis is in growing use in most of Europe, as well as in Australia, New Zealand, Mexico, South America, Asia, and the United States.

Iridology is the art and science of analyzing the color and structure of the iris of the eye to gain valuable health information. "Amazing" and "controversial" are two words often associated with it. It is both. It is amazing to all who see its wonders but do not yet perceive its secrets. It is controversial because of its struggle for acceptance by contemporary medicine as a valid examination method.

The story of modern iris analysis is the story of its discoverers and pioneers. Studying iridology is learning its philosophy of health and disease. It is taking the time to explore its territory, learn its unique landmarks, and practice its principles.

Iris analysis does not stand alone. It is part of a larger family. Its close relatives are the numerous branches of the natural and drugless healing arts. Its marriage partner is the art and science of nutrition, to which it is joined for all time.

If you have ever wondered about the secrets the iris can reveal, come with me now and explore. In Part One of this book, I will introduce you to iris analysis—its history, tools, language, and major signs. I will also explain, in layman's terms, how and why it works. In Part Two, I will help you put to use what you learned in Part One. Learn well, and enjoy the learning. You will not regret the time you put in, and you will use your new knowledge and skills forever.

Part One

Overview
of Iridology

*All cure starts from within out, from the head down, and in
the reverse order as the symptoms appeared.*

—Hering's Law of Cure

1.

The Big Picture

This story belongs to the eye. And we are going to let the eye tell it from its special point of view. The iris is a wonderful and colorful storyteller. By definition, the iris is that portion of the eye surrounding the pupil and giving the eye its distinctive color. It is the pigmentation of the iris that defines your baby blues or bashful browns. Since humans come equipped with a left and right iris, they possess one set of irides.

Iridology (i-rid-doll'-o-jee) is "the study of the iris, particularly of its color, markings, changes, etc., as associated with disease." This is according to the twenty-seventh edition of *Dorland's Illustrated Medical Dictionary.* The word "iris," like so many words in medicine, stems from the Greek and means "rainbow." Another translation is "halo." The iris surrounds the pupil of the eye and might easily be thought of as a kind of halo encircling it. More descriptively, however, it is a rainbow because of its color or colors.

The iris is the most distinctively colored portion of the eye. It is what we see in our mind when we think of a beautiful eye color. Your iris is your personal rainbow. The precept of iridology is that valuable information concerning a person's health and well-being can be obtained by studying this rainbow.

What irides reveal, and the fascinating way in which they relay the information, is the subject of this book.

It is very important to mention that information from the irides can be obtained quickly, painlessly, and inexpensively. That in itself ought to gain everyone's attention! Furthermore, a practitioner skilled in iris analysis can glean this information using nothing more than a simple, hand-held light source and a small magnifying lens. Expensive and complex equipment is not necessary to read an iris, although such apparatus is available for the serious, practicing iridologist and iridology researcher.

The practice of iridology is a covalent bond of science and art. Because iridology is practiced according to certain long-established and time-honored principles that constitute a rather well-defined and expanding body of knowledge, it rightly falls into the category of a science. At the same time, this fascinating science has some aspects of an art.

An iridologist must be able to exercise mental faculties that are not usually accessed through cold, scientific methodology. The iridologist's thinking must be broader. In keeping with the wholistic approach of iris analysis, the iridologist's attention must be focused on the person as much as on the person's complaints. Diseases can be dealt with scientifically; people are better dealt with artfully. Quality service to people seeks and employs the best of both dimensions, recognizing the unique value of each.

They say that there is nothing new under the sun. Maybe there isn't. But sometimes it takes a long time, even thousands of years, for people to *re*discover things. What they find may have been discovered before, but it surely is new to them. Such is the case with iridology. You may be surprised to learn that the idea of iridology, if not its practice, is nearly 2,000 years old, possibly even older. The idea is found in the Bible. Consider the verse in the sixth chapter of the book of St. Matthew. In verse twenty-two, we read, "The light of the body is the eye: if therefore thine eye be single, thy whole body shall be full of light." The Old English of the King James Version can be modernized to read, "The light of the body is the eye: so if your eye is pure, your whole body shall be full of light." Using iridology, we can see how the "purity," or "integrity," of the iris reflects the condition of tissues everywhere in the body.

You are now making your own discovery of iridology. For you, it is something new under the sun.

MEET DR. VON PECZELY AND REVEREND LILJEQUIST

Two European men who "rediscovered" the idea of iris analysis in the nineteenth century are generally considered today to share the title of "father of iridology." The first of these men is Dr. Ignatz von Peczely. (See Figure 1.1.) His is a story that may seem rather curious. However, bear in mind that it is not in the least unusual for the pacesetters of any era to say or do things that may seem bizarre or strange to those of a less inquiring mind.

It is interesting to note that nearly all traditions have a mythology. Iridology is no exception. Please remember that myths are not akin to fairy tales or fabrications, as many people erroneously believe. Myths are stories usually preserved through oral tradition for quite some time before being put to paper. Thus, their origins are often obscure and they do not always reflect the ultimate in historical accuracy. Nevertheless, they are built around a kernel of truth. Such is the case, I believe, with the story of Ignatz von Peczely and the owl.

Tradition holds that in 1837, Von Peczely, as a lad of about ten years of age, captured an owl in the family garden in Hungary. In an effort to escape from its captor's hand, the owl fractured its leg. Von Peczely claimed to notice immediately a spot that developed in the owl's iris at the 6:00 (six o'clock) position, which is to say the bottom part of the iris. We know from the iris chart (which we will discuss in Chapter 2) that this position corresponds to the leg. The iris mark made an impression on Von Peczely's young and inquisitive mind. Later in his life, Von Peczely noticed a similar marking in a man's iris. This sparked a remembrance of the encounter with the owl and brought the onset of the development of what is now modern iridology. Von Peczely went on to study medicine in Germany and later returned to his native Hungary to practice. He became quite well known as the doctor who could diagnose by looking into the eyes.

In recent years, it has been my privilege to meet and establish a friendship with Andre Peczely, who resides in San Mateo, California. When I met him, he had only an inkling of his Great Uncle Ignatz's work in iridology. He was surprised and pleased to learn of my work in this field and of the great esteem with which I hold his famous relative. Through his records and recollections of family life in Hungary, he has graciously provided me with much additional insight into the life of Dr. von Peczely. One of the unusual stories Andre Peczely told me was that Dr. von Peczely was an accomplished sculptor at the tender age of ten. Perhaps it was through this talent that he recognized something in the anatomical makeup of the eye that the average person usually misses.

The other father of iridology is Nils Liljequist, a Swedish clergyman who discovered iridology at about the same time as the young Von Peczely. (See Figure 1.2.) Liljequist's interest in the iris began around 1864 when he noticed in his own irides the appearance of discolorations. Through observation, he came to realize that such discolorations were associated with chemicals or drugs that were ingested or absorbed into the body. The observant clergyman noticed that each drug or chemical, however taken into the body, eventually resulted in a particular shade of discoloration in the iris.

The Swedish pastor eventually constructed what would develop into an elementary iris chart. The similarities between his drawings and those of Von Peczely are striking, especially since neither man at the time was familiar with the work of the other. Together, Dr. von Peczely and Reverend Liljequist are regarded as the founding fathers of the science and art of iridology as we have it today. These two iridology pioneers established themselves in about the year 1880.

LATER OUTSTANDING CONTRIBUTORS

Others, through the years, have also contributed to the development of iridology. Iridology was introduced in Germany largely through the work of Erdmann Leopold Stephanus Emanuel Felke, a clergyman who taught iridology to numerous students. Today in Germany, as a tribute to Pastor Felke's work, the Pastor Felke Institute is helping to develop and promote the

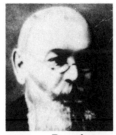

von Peczely,

Figure 1.1. Dr. Ignatz von Peczely became a father of iridology when he looked into the eyes of an owl that had just broken its leg. Von Peczely was ten years old at the time.

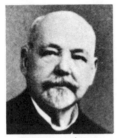

Liljequist

Figure 1.2. Reverand Nils Liljequist became the other father of iridology when he looked into his own eyes, which were discolored from drug accumulations.

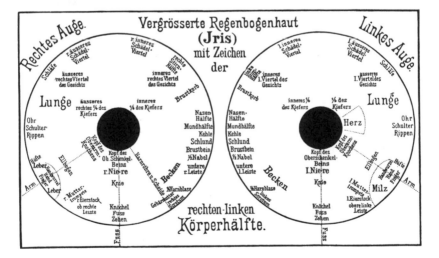

Figure 1.3. Dr. von Peczely and Reverend Liljequist developed iris charts that were strikingly similar even though neither man knew the other existed. The chart above is one of Von Peczely's first efforts, published in 1886 in the *Homeopatische Monatsblatter*.

science and art of iridology. Other German iridologists are Peter Johannes Theil, Josef Angerer, Theodor Kriege, and Josef Deck, to name but a few. Dr. Willie Hauser has now taken over for the late Dr. Deck.

From its birth in Hungary and incubation in Germany, iridology did not take long to break loose from its confinement on the European continent. By the turn of the century, it crossed the ocean and landed on the shores of its new frontier, North America. More than likely, the person responsible for the introduction of iridology to the United States was Henry Edward Lane, an Austrian medical doctor. He, in turn, taught Dr. Henry Lindlahr, a medical colleague, who spread the news of this new form of analysis through various publications. The publications included *Nature Cure*, a magazine, and *Iridiagnosis and Other Diagnostic Methods*, one book of a six-volume set published in 1919. Dr. Lindlahr had a profound effect on me.

Following my studies of the Lindlahr methods of analysis and nature healing, I spent time studying under Dr. R. M. McLain, a chiropractor and iridologist in Oakland, California. Another amongst the great American iridologists, Dr. John Dreier, of Glendale, California, also had a great influence on the development of iridology studies in America.

Still another name to mention in connection with the history of iridology is that of J. Haskel Kritzer, M.D. Dr. Kritzer wrote a textbook, *The Book of Iridiagnosis*, as well as developing one of the first iridology charts especially useful in teaching beginning students. Kritzer, like Liljequist before him, was deeply interested in the effects of drug accumulations in the body as observed in the iris. He was so taken with this idea that it became quite difficult for him to prescribe medications in his practice. Prescribing medications became an offense to his sense of ethics. He became increasingly interested in teaching "right living" in place of prescribing drugs to effect a cure.

In 1929, after reading the work of Kritzer and consulting with Dr. John Arnold, another California iridologist and the founder of the World Iridology Fellowship, I arranged to study with Dr. F. W. Collins, of Orange, New Jersey. With Dr. Collins, it was part of my work to sketch, in color, 500 irides of patients to point out the lesions and other markings germane to the study of iridology. This is a lesson that I still have not forgotten through my sixty-two years of iris analysis!

THE WORK CONTINUES

Despite its long and honorable history, iridology has had tough sledding. This emerging science has not been without its detractors and critics. Its arrival on American soil and continued pursuit of the mysteries resident in the iris fibers have proved to be anything but uneventful. Although it has advanced considerably, it sometimes has been the subject of harsh criticism. Probably because of, and certainly in spite of, this criticism, iridology and its practice have gained new strength.

Although a number of persons in the United States have taken up iridology, written books about it, and spent time lecturing and teaching, I believe I have spent more time, and delved into the subject deeper, than anyone. I feel as though I have been driven to iridology by powerful forces deep within me. Nearly all of the profits I have made over the years have been plowed back into my iridology work.

I entered the private practice of chiropractic in 1929. However, I found that most of my patients needed not only my chiropractic services, but also lessons on how to live right, how to garden, how to select foods, and how to devise a menu for their family. They needed to learn how to correctly prepare and cook their food. We all know that old habits die hard. My patients needed to be taught how to obtain the best for themselves so they could get well and stay well. But I found that I could not spend enough time with each one of them to teach them all the things they needed. So, in 1931, I established my first sanitarium. In sanitarium-style living, I had access to my patients on a daily basis. We lived together. I taught them how to break old habits and put new ones in their place. And, out with the old habits went the old health complaints. You see, proper living results in robust health. Poor living habits bring fatigue, sickness, and unhappiness.

I'm mentioning my years of sanitarium experience because during all those years, iridology was my guide and stay. I became known as the doctor who looked into your eyes and then told you what you had to do to improve your health. During those years, I had people from all over the world come to my sanitarium in search of better health. And I looked in the eyes of each and every one of them. In fact, I have looked into more than 300,000 eyes in my sixty-two years of practice! These irides told me what each person needed in his life. They were my guide to suggesting the proper treatment, exercise, and diet. Through this work, I saw the results of iridology.

After experiencing my success with iridology, I began to think that it would be wonderful if more people knew how to take advantage of this science. Average people would then have a philosophical background to help them better understand their bodies. They would learn about the unity of disease and know better how to care for the body nutritionally and closer to the laws of nature, as we were intended to. I, therefore, began to teach classes in iridology and nutrition. My thought from the first was to teach anyone who wanted to learn: laypersons from all walks of life and health professionals as well. Before long, I was teaching these classes in various parts of the world.

After more than forty-five years in sanitarium practice, I sold my last sanitarium, Hidden Valley Ranch, in Escondido, California, in 1976. I decided to devote my remaining years to iridology and nutrition research, teaching, and writing. I have published numerous books during my years, including the culmination of my life's work in iridology, *Iridology: The Science and Practice in the Healing Arts, Volume II.* First published in 1982, it is an update of my very first text on the subject, *The Science and Practice of Iridology,* which I published way back in 1952. The preliminary book is still around today and is now in its twelfth printing.

On a recent trip to China, I was greatly surprised to find that the Chinese had translated several of my books, including my first iridology text. I found that I had quite a following in China of my work in iridology and nutrition. Although I am continuing my heavy schedule of teaching and writing, my interest of late has been learning how to utilize the speed and accuracy of the modern computer to help analyze the iris. I will further discuss my work with computers later in this book.

IRIDOLOGY AND THE WHOLISTIC PRINCIPLE

People are talking a lot these days about wholistic healing. Practitioners engaged in wholistic healing take into consideration the whole person. They don't just treat disease; they treat people. This philosophy recognizes that the pain in your neck may be your boss at work. Wholism considers the importance of the 99 percent of you on the other end of your injured finger. It affirms that your wholeness is something more than just the sum of your discrete parts. It says that you are more than just a body within which may be residing a disease.

Those who embrace the wholistic concept are more apt to consider the person, as opposed to merely his disease. The cart must not be placed before the horse. Diseases do not create people; it is people who create disease. We need to affirm that we don't *catch* diseases. *We create them by breaking down our natural defenses through the way we eat, drink, think, and live.* There is a saying that all disease can be cured, but not all people. The emphasis must be on the person, not on the disease. Dead people can't be cured of anything. It is wholistic thinking that is willing to consider the meaning resident in the words, "The light of the body is the eye. . . ." Iris analysis belongs with wholistic health care.

The iridologist is a wholistic thinker when it comes to considerations of health. It is the iridologist who looks to the iris of the eye and sees that, indeed, the eye is the light of the body. And to the degree that the iris is healthy, whole, single, pure, and perfect, the health of the body will be too.

"The Enlightened One" is a title that has been given to various figures in history. These people have usually led pure, simple, and exemplary lives. They have "seen the light." Iridology is a method of putting light in dark places. Darkness is associated with evil and the impure, while light is associated with goodness and purity. Everyone desires to be enlightened, to see, to know, and to understand. Iridology is a means of gaining understanding and becoming enlightened about the body. It is for discovering the dark places and bringing light to them. It is not enough to be a doctor. It is better to be a healer.

Sometimes iridology seems almost too good to be true. It is said that if something sounds too good to be true, it probably is. We must be careful. Iridology can't tell everything about a person's health. No method of health analysis, whatever its means, is perfect. It is best to beware of exaggerated claims. Like other methods, iris analysis has its limitations. And within these limitations, its unique value can be properly defined. What iris analysis is and how you can use it to improve your health and avoid disease are what we are about to look into.

YOUR EYES REVEAL THE REAL YOU

Even the casual observer will notice that the iris appears to be less than homogenous in its appearance. Both its color and structure vary markedly from person to person and even from right eye to left eye in the same individual. What romantic fails to notice eye color or the sensual allure of pupils dilated in sympathetic acceptance of amorous advances? We have all experienced glaring eyes, soulful eyes, wandering eyes, fearful eyes, and even tearful eyes. But have you ever heard of the skin, the bones, or the blood described with similar expressions?

The eyes are the most expressive organs in the body. Nowadays, we have the ability to dress our eyes in various colors through the use of tinted contact lenses. We can make fashion statements with our eyeglass frames, cosmetics, and accessories.

One of the first things people notice is the eyes. We communicate through the appearance and use of our eyes. A good speaker makes frequent eye contact with his listeners. An old song is "Speak to Me Only With Thine Eyes." One person can have an eye for beauty, while another has an eye for a bargain. You will see what you are on the lookout for. Truly, the eyes are revealing. Sometimes the lips may be saying "no," but the eyes are saying "yes"!

The eyes communicate in a special way for the iridologist. Iris color, structure, and special markings are interpreted by the practitioner to attain valuable information about the patient as a whole. Iris analysis is about communication. Your body communicates with the iridologist using the iris as the vehicle of transmission. There is possibly more truth than we realize in the saying that the eye is the most complicated tissue in the whole body.

There are a number of special studies of the eye that concern themselves with areas other than the iris. Let's now consider some of these. They can help define iridology by indicating what it is not.

WHAT IRIDOLOGY IS NOT

Perhaps the best known medical discipline dealing with the eye is ophthalmology. But iridology is not ophthalmology. Ophthalmology is the branch of allopathic medicine that deals with diseases and dysfunction of the eye. Allopathic medicine is the branch of medicine that treats disease utilizing drugs and surgery. An ophthalmologist is an allopathic medical specialist. As a physician, he treats disease and dysfunction. Drugs and surgery are his most common prescriptions.

Ophthalmologists can also examine for, and prescribe, corrective lenses, although optometrists are increasingly assuming this aspect of eye care. It is not the function of the iridologist to examine the eyes per se for disease or dysfunction. However, the astute lay practitioner, as well as the professional iridologist, should always refer a client for further examination and appropriate care when necessary or when in doubt.

Neither ophthalmology nor iridology should be confused with optometry. Iridology is not optometry. Optometry is the branch of medicine that concerns itself primarily with the examination for, and correction of, refractive errors of vision utilizing optical lenses. Complementary to the optometrist is the optician, who specializes in dispensing the lenses and associated eyewear prescribed by the ophthalmologist or optometrist. Neither of these professionals is associated with iridology, nor do they use the analysis techniques of the iridologist.

Optometrists, as well as many other specialists and general practitioners, use a tool called the "ophthalmoscope" to focus a bright light in the eye. Nearly everyone has had this examination. This simple procedure allows visualization of the retina, which is the part of the eye that changes light waves into electrical impulses. These impulses are then transmitted directly to the brain by the optic nerve. The brain interprets them, and this special interpretation is what we experience as sight.

An ophthalmoscopic examination is extremely useful for detecting early manifestations of quite a number of diseases and conditions. It provides the doctor with a great deal of useful health information. Its use should not be underestimated, but at the same time, it should be remembered that this procedure is not associated with iridology and does not share the same principles.

Besides these orthodox health-care practices dealing with the eye, there are a number of lesser known practices that embody the study of the eye. One that is sometimes confused with iridology is sclerology. The sclera is the white of the eye and does not include the iris. People who perform an analysis of the sclera are known as "sclerologists." Like iridologists, sclerologists seek to interpret the color, markings, and topography of the eye, but in contrast to the iridologist's concentration on the iris, the sclerologist fixes his attention on the sclera.

One of the things iridologists and sclerologists have in common is that they both seek to only interpret physical signs in the eye. They do not, nor should they, make their examination for the purpose of diagnosing disease. Nor is their concern with refractive errors of vision or with treatment of the eye. Their expertise is confined exclusively to observation and interpretation.

ANALYSIS PREFERRED TO DIAGNOSIS

A number of early iridologists referred to their work as either "iridiagnosis" or "irisdiagnosis." Latter-day iridologists refer to the examination of the iris as "iris analysis." In recent years, I have chosen to use the term "neuroptic analysis" to define my work with the iris. Nowadays, nearly all iridologists have turned to the term "analysis," forsaking the use of "diagnosis." This change in terminology has come about partly to avoid running afoul of the law. We need to examine the meaning of these terms in order to understand what lies ahead.

In the United States, making a diagnosis implies that you are a doctor duly licensed to engage in diagnostic function. This function usually is either the naming of a disease or the declaration of health. It is well to keep in mind that not even all registered health practitioners can legally diagnose disease. For example, although a registered, duly licensed physical therapist can engage in the activity of providing physical therapy, he cannot legally make a diagnosis.

The making of a diagnosis is reserved only for doctors. Since quite a number of persons who engage in iris analysis are not registered and licensed doctors, they cannot legally make a diagnosis. The term "analysis" does not have such an explicit legal definition. Thus, it is the term of choice of iridologists and the one most often used by them. It is essential for the survival and promotion of iridology that those who choose to engage in its practice avoid naming any disease condition. As we have seen, to do so is to infringe on rights reserved exclusively for doctors and can land the iridologist, sooner or later, in a snarl of legal troubles.

Not only is it not permissible from a legal standpoint to name disease from examination of the iris, but in truth, iris analysis does not lend itself to the discernment of disease per se. There are no iris markings or colors of which I am aware that are uniquely and unerringly associated with a particular disease state. There is the Kayser-Fleischer ring, a golden-brown or gray-green pigment deposit where the cornea meets the iris, which is associated with Wilson's disease. It could be thought of as an iris sign due to its proximity to that structure, but it is actually the discoloration of a membrane contiguous with, and confined to, the cornea, not the iris. When manifest, however, it is a reliable indicator of the condition. Wilson's disease is a familial disorder of copper metabolism. A familial disease is one that tends to run in a family but is not a genetic disorder because it does not follow the strict rules of genetic determination. Diabetes is probably the most common familial disease. It is a familial tendency rather than a genetic certainty.

It is better for the iridologist to refrain from suggesting to a person that he has any particular disease, letting such diagnostics remain the province of licensed doctors. In so doing, the iridologist will avoid transgressing the law and stepping on the toes of those who are legally qualified to diagnose. He will also keep from creating what may prove to be false hopes or fears in those he analyzes. Every doctor knows that an error in diagnosis can be worse than no diagnosis at all. Therefore, we must be very careful in our iris work to never name a disease or give any information that may be construed as diagnostic. By definition, iris analysis is: *To discern by observation of the irides the various stages of tissue inflammation—acute, subacute, chronic, and degenerative—and where the inflammations are located. Inherent weaknesses and their locations can also be discerned.*

It is indeed unfortunate that one of the greatest pitfalls awaiting the iridologist is the temptation to name diseases. The feelings of satisfaction and power resulting from conferring a name are deeply rooted in the human psyche. For example, the Bible tells us that man's first task on Earth was to name the animals, thus giving him power and dominion over them. The children's fairy tale of Rumpelstiltskin illustrates man's struggle to break the spell that ignorance imposes and gain the freedom and control that come with being able to call an adversary by name.

Strong is the temptation to name diseases because nearly everyone has come to expect that his malady has a name. Patients have come to expect, and doctors have been trained to make, a diagnosis. "Diagnosis" comes from the Greek and means "through knowledge." Since no one wants an ignorant doctor, patients expect that through his knowledge, the physician will display his mastership of a disease by giving it a label. If the doctor can't do this, the patient may become *im*patient and seek a doctor who can. "After all," the patient may reason, "how can you hope to deal with my condition if you aren't knowledgeable enough to call it by name?"

There is no magic in the reading of an iris. There is no flag popping up in the iris bearing the name of a disease. Naming and classifying a disease and making an intelligent and knowledgeable diagnosis are very difficult and challenging endeavors for any doctor. But merely attaching a name, however sophisticated that name may be, does not effect a cure.

Since the iridologist truly cannot name any disease by merely observing the iris, he must employ a different way of communicating what he learns from the halo of the eye. The best way to do this is to use the specific terminology developed by iridologists that can help to better relate the information gleaned from the iris. By using this new terminology, you will discover that it is not necessary to name diseases in order to exercise dominion over them. The new terminology will also help you to understand how to truly reverse the progression of disease since it will help you to learn from the iris how disease and ill health are developed.

These, then, are two of my goals for this book: to introduce you to the terminology used by iridologists and to show you how to apply it. We will begin this in the next chapter. This book is not meant to be a medical book or a bible, just a guide. Use it like a road map. And please enjoy your trip!

2.

There's More to Iridology Than Meets the Eye

Since Ignatz von Peczely first looked into the injured owl's eyes with nothing but his own bare eyes about 150 years ago, iridology has developed into an exacting science utilizing a specific terminology and tools. This chapter will discuss the most important and commonly used tools and terms, including the fascinating iris chart. Additional terminology will be presented throughout the rest of the book.

THE IRIS CHART

One of the most interesting aspects of iridology is the iris chart. The iris chart shows the areas in the iris that correspond to the different parts of the body. For an example, take a look at Figure 2.1, which presents the Jensen chart.

The first thing to observe on the Jensen chart is that although the right and left irides are similar, they are not identical. The map of the right iris is at the reader's left, whereas the map of the left iris is at the reader's right. This is so the chart can be used to read the irides of another person. The mirror-image chart shown in Figure 2.2 should be used for reading your own irides.

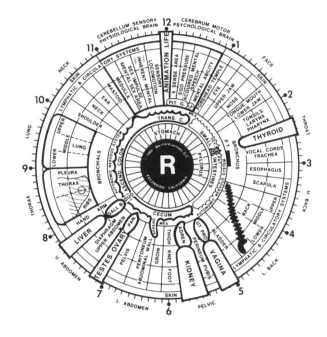

Figure 2.1. The modern Jensen iris chart should be used when examining the irides of another person. Note how the left and right irides are similar but not identical.

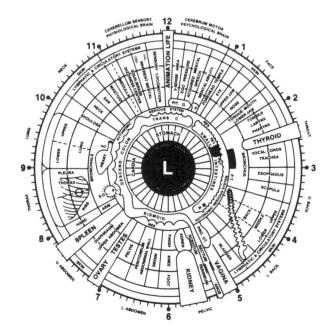

Figure 2.2. The reverse Jensen iris chart should be used when examining your own eyes. It corresponds to what you would see if you looked at your eyes in a mirror.

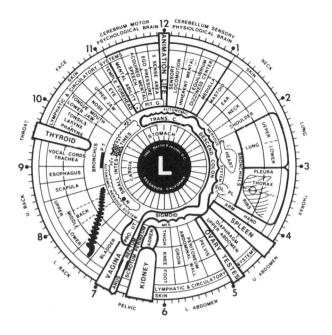

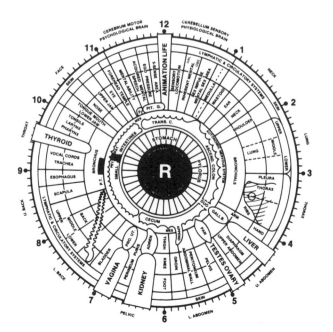

There are 166 named areas in the iris chart, with 80 in the right iris and 86 in the left iris. These do not include the areas immediately outside the circular periphery of the right and left maps, which indicate more generalized locations. If the chart seems rather complex and detailed, please keep in mind that early charts were much simpler. The present charts used by iridologists reflect many years of development in the science of iris analysis. You can see how the chart evolved by comparing the latest Jensen chart to the early iris chart in Figure 1.3 on page 9. Comparing this historical German chart with the latest Jensen chart, the greater detail of the latter is striking.

A cursory examination of the Jensen chart will reveal that the brain areas extend from the 11:00 (eleven o'clock) position to the 1:00 (one o'clock) position. Most iridologists find it convenient to think of the iris and its chart as resembling a clock face for the purpose of easily locating specific areas. Correspondingly, the lungs and chest area are at 3:00 on the left iris (9:00 in the right), and the legs and feet are straight down at 6:00.

Notice too that the areas are arranged in both a circular pattern and a radial pattern. In other words, the chart is comprised of a number of concentric circles that are further divided into several more or less pie-shaped slices. Some people prefer to think of the chart as resembling a wheel, with the pupil as the hub and most of the areas resembling spokes. This is also a useful comparison.

There is no perfect graphic analogy to the chart's construction since it is somewhat asymetrical and deviates from any regimental pattern that might be artificially imposed. Nevertheless, even the casual observer should notice that the chart does generally conform to a recognizable geometric pattern and is not of unorganized or haphazard construction. This is extremely important because the practicing and competent iridologist must be able to see in the chart's construction a highly evolved graphic depiction of the relationship that the body organs and systems have to one another. Please notice, for example, that the foot is at the 6:00 position, at the bottom of the chart. Notice also that the brain areas are at the top portion of the chart. The lungs and pleura (the sacs that enclose the lungs) reside horizontally on the outside, as opposed to the inside, or nasal side, of the chart. Continued observation will affirm that

the chart layout conforms generally with the anatomical place-
ment of the body organs and structures. (See Figure 2.3.)

The Charted Iris Zones

There is another aspect of the iris chart that deserves mention.
This is the division of the chart into so-called "zones." Some
iridologists ascribe greater importance to these zoned areas than
do others. Frankly, I have never thought to place too much
importance on them. Some iridologists claim that one zone
represents the inside of hollow organs while another zone represents the outside of these structures. I would not argue that
this isn't true, but I do feel that these ideas are better left to the

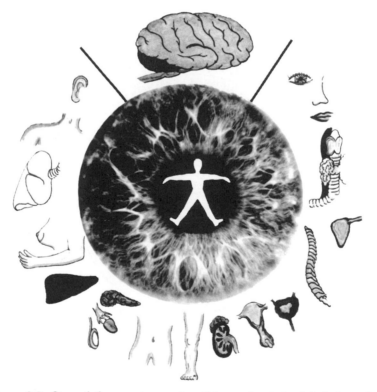

Figure 2.3. One of the most amazing things about the iris is how its
arrangement corresponds to the body. For example, the brain areas are
represented at the top while the feet are at the bottom, and the bowel
area is on the inside while the skin is on the outside.

experienced iridologist. They are beyond the scope of this iridology primer.

With few exceptions, I find that in practice, iris zones are rather ill-defined. Most simply do not have the perfectly circumscribed borders assigned to them in the charts. I do not mean to imply that zones are not useful in providing a generalized location. I do believe, however, that they are best considered to be a guide, an approximation.

There are seven zones that have been empirically imposed upon the iris chart. I will draw attention to these zones as we deal with certain iris signs that lay more or less within them. Figure 2.4 presents a chart of the seven zones.

Now that we have a basic idea of how the iris chart is constructed, let's take a look at the tools used by the iridologist.

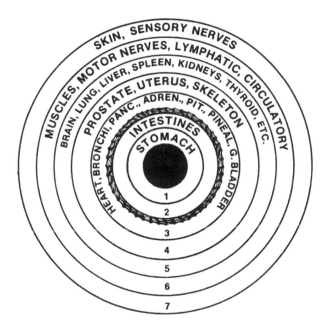

Figure 2.4. Many iridologists also divide the iris into zones, which form concentric circles within the chart. I use seven zones, but I use them as an aid to locating signs only.

TOOLS USED IN IRIS ANALYSIS

By far the greatest tool anyone has is his mind. Since iridology is an interpretive art as well as a science, we must use our mental facilities carefully. It is this subjectivity of interpretation that makes iridology an art. In the future, iridology will become less subjective in nature as computers increasingly provide a level of objectivity that was impossible before their advent. More later on the role of computers in iridology.

Due to their small size and relative intricacy, magnifying lenses quickly became the common tool that iridologists use to view the iris. (See Figure 2.5.) Iridologists have experimented with a wide variety of lenses and optical devices in an effort to better see the tiny fibers that constitute the iris structure. The same as the practitioners of any developing science, people in the field of iridology are constantly engaged in an effort to find the perfect method for observing the iris. I suggest using a hand-held magnifying glass of superior-quality optics and utilizing "4×" power. A glass of less power doesn't provide enough magnification to visualize the fibers well. A glass of poorer quality exhibits increasing distortion as its periphery is approached and sometimes distorts color as well. There are iridologists who prefer to work with lenses much stronger than 4×, but I find this magnification to be adequate.

In the quest for ever-better visualization of the iris, iridologists have experimented with the tools of ophthalmology, such as the ophthalmoscope, slit-lamp, and other devices of illumination and magnification. There is no doubt that such devices are useful, but most are not ideally suited to iridology and are best reserved for advanced students and researchers.

In addition to magnification, adequate illumination is also necessary for obtaining a good view of the iris. Early iridologists simply viewed the iris with the naked eye, using natural sunlight for illumination. Dr. F. W. Collins, of East Orange, New Jersey, one of my best teachers, preferred sunlight above any other form of illumination. Although sunlight can provide excellent illumination with true color rendition, it may not always be convenient to get or available when needed.

Perhaps the best alternative to sunlight is the common flashlight. (See Figure 2.5 again.) It can be purchased nearly anywhere and is convenient, inexpensive, easy to use, and very adequate. When purchasing a flashlight for iris analysis, be sure it is either pre-focused or can be focused to a bright spot. To check, simply shine the light on a wall. The chances are that the light will either be focused to a bright spot or will be diffused like a floodlight. Some lights shine in a ring of light. Neither this latter type nor a diffused light is acceptable. Another type of light allows the user to focus the beam. This type is acceptable if it can be focused easily to a spot. Some lights have a halogen or krypton lamp, both of which provide a whiter and brighter illumination. Although helpful, this extra brightness is not essential.

The various techniques of iris illumination could be a study in themselves. In my over sixty-two years of iris analysis, I have devised and used many tools. However, I find myself always returning to the simplicity and effectiveness of the pre-focused flashlight and hand-held 4× magnifying glass.

Sunlight or a flashlight plus a hand-held magnifier provide good clarity and definition for viewing the iris. But this method has the disadvantage of being tedious for both the subject and iridologist. Neither the subject nor the examiner should be required to maintain one position for an extended period. Also, subjects tire quickly of a bright light shining into their eyes, even for brief periods. In addition to these discomforts, there is no adequate way for the iridologist to make an accurate and permanent record of what he sees. He must rely on his power of recall.

Early iridologists attempted to make a crude sketch of the iris as they peered into the eye with their glass. In earlier days, I sketched many an iris just this way, using colored pencils to lend life and accuracy to my work. You will recall that Dr. Collins had me sketch 500 irides using colored pencils before I graduated as an iridologist. I learned iridology the hard way!

Early in my professional development, I began to experiment with various types of photographic equipment. I wanted to see if I could assemble camera equipment that would take an adequate picture of the iris. With the introduction of color film and more sophisticated technology, iris photography eventually came into its own. With a photograph, an iridologist can examine an iris carefully and without strain. No longer is the subject required to sit uncomfortably still for more than the few seconds needed to snap a set of pictures. Gone is the feeling of being pressed for time in making the analysis as the iris can now be examined at the leisure and convenience of the iridologist. These and other advantages of iris photography are a giant step forward.

For many years, iridologists had no commercial apparatus available that was designed especially for their use. Those desiring iris photos were compelled to improvise, using whatever items were available. Some iridologists were quite innovative. In my personal quest for the perfect iris photo, I frequently had to have certain elements specially designed and fabricated, a costly and time-consuming venture. Necessity being the mother of invention, years of experimentation gave birth to a series of original designs. However, although some proved to be quite good, I was never entirely satisfied.

My quest for ever-better iris photos eventually culminated with the Jensen Iriscope, as it is called. (See Figure 2.6.) I believe this camera is the finest apparatus assembled expressly for iris photography. The many years and countless hours devoted to the perfection of this photographic equipment have resulted in a camera that takes excellent-quality transparencies of the iris. The new professional films give excellent color rendition. A special lens designed and ground to conform to the curved surface of the iris virtually eliminates optical distortion. And fiberoptic and angled side-lighting assures safety as well as an enhanced perception of depth-of-field. The special lens and lighting make the difference and set this camera apart from any other.

In addition to the camera, a zoom microscope attachment is available. (See Figure 2.6 again.) This device allows binocular viewing of the iris, incorporating the advantage of continuously variable magnification. I believe this is the best equipment the serious iridologist can have for practice as well as research purposes.

Iridologists have found through experimentation that the best way to view the photograph of an iris is as a projected color transparency. Transparencies (slides) have better color rendition

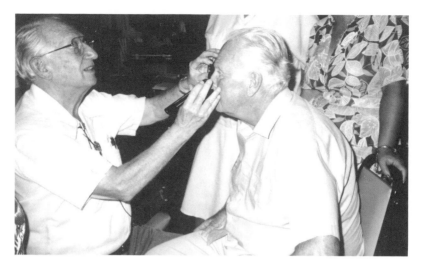

Figure 2.5. In October 1988, I conducted an iridology class during which I had the pleasure of examining the eyes of Andre Peczely, a great nephew of Dr. Ignatz von Peczely. I used a hand-held 4X magnifying glass and common flashlight.

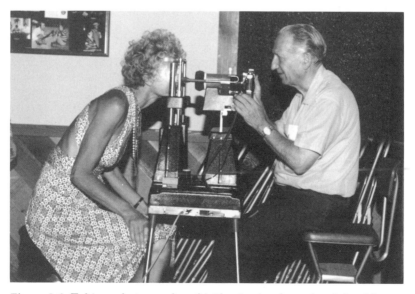

Figure 2.6. Taking photographs of irides is simple and quick with my Jensen Iriscope, the finest equipment for iris photography assembled to date. Note the camera with its special lens, angled side-lighting, and zoom microscope attachment.

and definition than do paper prints, which are subject to more variations in exposure and dyes. Also, prints are subject to more color fading with age than are transparencies.

Transparent grids have been developed, at first directly from the iris chart, for overlaying on the projected image to ensure accuracy in the location of the chart areas. To facilitate further accuracy, projection zoom lenses with continuously variable focal lengths enabled the projected iris image to very closely approximate the grid. However, the grids have now been modified to closer approximate the natural, slightly elliptical shape of the iris. (See Figure 2.7.) Also modified were the colon areas of the chart to correspond better with what is shown on the iris slides. Iridologists refer to these new grids as an "amorphous grid" design. The grids represent a slight departure from the more stylized iris chart and have become the standard grid used with projected color transparencies.

As with the camera, my associates and I pursued many avenues in our quest for improved methods for viewing iris slides. We tried various types of projection and viewing devices. The best arrangement we have found so far involves dual 35-millimeter slide projectors, each equipped with a zoom lens. (See Figure 2.8.) The iris images are focused on rear projection screens, placed about five-and-a-half feet away. The right and left grids are then attached as overlays onto the front of the screens, using masking tape.

One of the invaluable features of this equipment is that the viewer can change slides and focus them by remote control. This allows the iridologist to remain seated while viewing both irides or when doing comparison work. Most analysis work is done using a projected iris diameter of about five to eight inches. For teaching purposes, I sometimes use screens that are large enough to display irides with a diameter of about one-and-a-half feet.

A NEW LANGUAGE FOR IRIDOLOGY

In addition to special tools, every science also has its own particular language, its terminology. And to understand the terminology is to understand the science. The language of iridology is centered around tissue integrity.

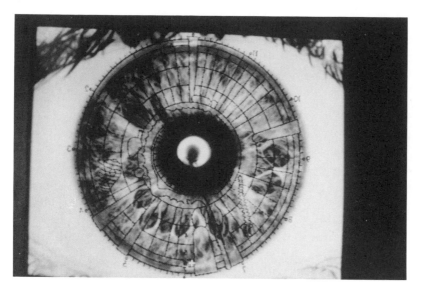

Figure 2.7. A grid laid over the projected photographic image of an iris helps the iridologist to locate specific chart areas. Today's grids use an amorphous design.

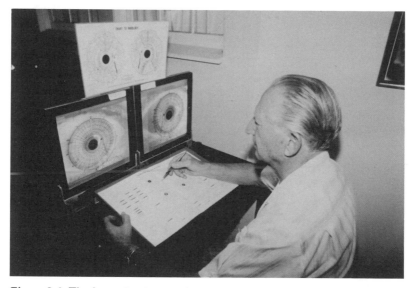

Figure 2.8. The best viewing equipment we have developed so far involves dual 35-millimeter slide projectors, equipped with zoom lenses, and rear projection screens. The slides are changed by remote control.

What an iris analysis seeks to carefully discern is the integrity of remote tissues in the body as represented by the structure, color, and density of the minute fibers of the iris. As we will see in Chapter 4, this is possible due to the presence of established nerve pathways in the body that conduct nerve impulses from every location to the brain and then to the iris. This happens because the eye is an anatomical extension of the brain.

A long-established physiological axiom holds that illness usually begins with some type of overactivity, which is an acuteness in the tissues. If left untreated, this condition either will resolve or will progress in time to a chronic and underactive state. Also, overactive tissues or conditions that are receiving inappropriate therapy, which is treatment that is not in accordance with nature's principles, will progress in time to a chronic and underactive state.

Long-term chronic conditions of underactivity will cause ever-diminishing cellular activity, with the affected tissues finally becoming degenerative and nonfunctional. Iridologists refer to this process as "tissue degeneration." Medical doctors also recognize this condition as degenerative, with their so-called "chronic degenerative diseases" being those diseases in which certain tissues are in a state of underactivity. This is the type of condition in which the number of sufferers is growing. It is also the type of condition for which medicine no longer holds out much hope for a cure but prefers instead to focus on long-term management. These are the diseases with which we are told we must learn to live.

Arthritis, cardiovascular disease, and cancer are all chronic degenerative diseases. What's more, they are immediately recognized as three of the worst health problems affecting the Western World. With cancer, the tissues are in an altered state of energy. With all of them, tissues are dying or in a state of extremely low energy. I like to think of these states of activity— acute, chronic, and degenerative—as representing a tissue's integrity.

A tissue with a normal amount of energy, and thus of high integrity, is neither overactive (acute) nor underactive (chronic). It is somewhere in-between and just right. This is the balance of health: not too much and not too little. Doctors call this balanced condition "homeostasis." When we are homeostatic, we feel wonderful. It has become my custom to begin my lectures by saying, "I feel wonderful! How do you feel?" When you have good tissue integrity, you can joyfully respond in kind.

Iris analysis concerns itself with tissue integrity, not with diagnosed conditions or named diseases. Always remember that there can be no degenerative disease process without a corresponding alteration in tissue integrity. If you adhere to this central idea, you will not stray from the central precept of iris analysis: *The art and science of iridology is the evaluation of tissue integrity, including inherent strengths and weaknesses, collectively called "constitution."*

Iridologists use the word "integrity" when referring to tissue the same way anyone would use the word. It is common to speak of a person as having integrity and even of inanimate things as possessing integrity. It's a good word. It conveys wholeness, inclusiveness, firmness, fine construction, flawlessness, health, well-being, security, and honesty.

You will find it easier to gain a working knowledge of iris analysis and an appreciation of its concepts if you look at tissues with the thought of evaluating their integrity. If you can train yourself to think in this manner, you can stay away from attempts to name and classify disease. After all, perfect tissue integrity can have no disease associated with it. Only when tissue integrity is somehow compromised or overwhelmed can disease gain a foothold. Evaluating tissue integrity is the proper work of the iridologist when making an iris analysis.

Through iridology, you will find that many conditions can affect tissue integrity. Changes in climate and altitude, changes in blood circulation and blood pressure, chemical deficiencies and excesses, toxic settlements, inherent weaknesses, glandular imbalances, metabolic upsets, oxygenation of the blood, trauma, and psychosomatic influences—to name but a few—can alter tissue integrity. Iris analysis is the assessment of tissue integrity.

Before we continue our study of the iris and how to evaluate the integrity of the tissues it represents, we need to digress for a moment and attend to an important matter. It is said that there is nothing as powerful as the imagination. Making an evaluation of tissues represented in the iris can have a powerful effect on the mind. Many a student of medicine, reading through books describing the symptoms of a disease, has ascribed the symptoms to himself. When I was a young student studying the medical books, I thought that I had the symptoms of nearly every rare disease I read about. It's easy for the imagination to run wild. I hope you won't have this experience as you learn to evaluate the iris. The mere presence of less-than-perfect iris signs is not in itself an indication that a person is afflicted with some terrible condition. Remember, no individual is in perfect health. As beautifully constructed as we are, we all fall short of physical perfection.

Another popular saying claims that a little knowledge is a dangerous thing. This certainly applies to iridology. The well-trained and experienced iridologist does not become upset over what he sees in the iris. The prudent iridologist is especially careful about how he tells a client what he has visualized and the meaning that it may hold. Students must be especially aware that people can be easily frightened and misled, not only by *what* is said by the examiner but also by *how* it is said. Few conditions are as serious as they seem. Many are not serious at all and only need a little attention. Remember, the iris is a sensitive instrument and often reveals what we call "preclinical" conditions. These can be minor tissue alterations that will manifest themselves in symptoms only if left ignored. They sometimes require years to reach the point where symptoms really do occur.

The best way for the beginning student to learn is to ask the subject if he is having any trouble in the areas that may be revealing a problem. If there is a history of problems, make note of it. If problems in the area are denied, make note of this also. Often, the same person, seen at a later date, sometimes even after years, admits to having had some trouble in the area during the time since his last visit. This is an education for the iridologist. After practicing for sixty-two years and analyzing over 300,000 irides, I am still very careful about what I say to a person. I much prefer to *ask* about the things I see rather than *tell* too much. You see, I am still a student!

You, like everyone else, are going to leave this world when your time comes. Be careful you don't hasten that time for another person because of what you say to him. It is a fact that many people worry themselves into ill health. Be careful not to plant destructive seeds of worry in a subject's mind. Some people can "worry themselves to death." Be wise, prudent, and tactful.

3.

Look Into
My Eyes

We have learned what iris analysis is and what it is not. We have also reviewed what kind of equipment is best and how to get set up to examine the iris. We've discussed some terminology. Now let's continue by taking an actual look into our eyes, or perhaps the irides of a family member or friend. The purpose here is not to engage in an in-depth study of iridology, but to learn enough essentials to be able to demonstrate its value to ourselves. Let's begin our investigation with iris color.

IRIS COLOR

Iridologists say that nearly all eyes are either basically blue or basically brown. Historically persons coming from the warmer and equatorial zones of the Earth have brown eyes and those from the more temperate and colder regions have blue eyes. Nowadays, of course, our planet is very cosmopolitan. Because of this, and from all the intermarriage between the races, we now find blue, brown, and various mixtures of the two almost all over the globe. In addition, iris color can also be influenced by drug accumulations and toxic chemical settlements in the body. We will discuss these later.

If you can distinctly see the tiny, and more or less wavy, white or perhaps slightly yellow lines extending radially from the pupil margin to near the periphery of the iris, then you likely have a basically blue eye, even if it appears to be another color. The color can appear light or dark blue, perhaps even light to moderate brown. You may even think it has a slight greenish tint. If the irides are more on the brown side, you may think that you indeed have brown eyes. But the experiences iridologist will know that from a heredity standpoint, if you can distinctly discern the individual iris fibers, your eyes are more blue than brown.

By contrast, a genuine brown iris—as commonly visualized in Mexican, Negroid, Oriental, and Mediterranean people, for example—is very brown, sometimes even quite muddy brown in appearance. In dark brown irides, the thin fibers are difficult or impossible to discern distinctly. This isn't due to some major difference in anatomical construction, but rather because of the underlying brown pigment in the iris. If heavy, the pigment can obscure the individual fibers that are easily seen in the basically blue iris. When nearly all the iris fibers are obscured and the iris appears brown, there is little doubt that the iris really is a true brown. Frequently, blue eyes are mistaken for brown, but almost never vice versa.

Some irides defy the inexperienced iridologist to label them either basically brown or basically blue. Iridologists usually refer to these irides as "mixed." I often refer to a basically blue iris exhibiting a brown hue as a "blue mix," or simply as "mixed." For an example of a mixed iris, as well as of blue and brown irides, please see Figure 3.2.

Blue irides are generally easier to analyze than brown irides because the iris fibers are more distinct. The absence of heavy, dark pigmentation makes viewing easier. With experience, however, even heavily pigmented dark brown eyes can be analyzed well. Still, some things remain that cannot be seen as well in dark irides as in lighter ones. Therefore, we are looking to the computer to aid in better analyzing dark brown eyes. More about computers later.

If you are a beginner, you will find it easier to start by

looking at light eyes. Then, after gaining more confidence in your examinations, you can progress to examining darker irides. Very dark brown irides require brighter illumination and more than a little experience to analyze well. Practice first by trying to determine whether the iris color is blue, brown, or mixed.

CONSTITUTION

"Constitution" is a term used by the iridologist to indicate the qualitative and quantitative stuff of which we are biologically made. It is our physical makeup, our genetic gift, received and perhaps to be bestowed. I might say that no one comes into the world with a perfect constitution. I don't know anyone who is physically perfect. Everyone falls short of perfection from a constitution standpoint. All people have areas of relative inherent strength, as well as of weakness. By "relative," I mean, for example, a kidney that is inherently weak when compared with a lung that is inherently stronger. Even the mythical Achilles had his heel. Some people, however, are stronger overall than are others.

It is most tempting for the beginner in iridology to think of stronger as better and weaker as less desirable. But, as we shall see, this is not necessarily so. Inherent strengths and weaknesses are also relative in the sense that that's where you get them from—your relatives.

Constitution is often illustrated by comparing a piece of furniture crafted out of pine to a piece constructed from oak. Pine is a soft, loose-grained wood. Oak, on the other hand, exhibits a harder, more tightly grained growth. Both are beautiful, but oak can take more misuse than pine can. The pine piece needs more care to keep it functional and looking good. It cannot take the same punishment as oak. This difference in the structure of wood can represent constitution as seen in the iris. People with weak constitutions need to concentrate more on their health requirements in order to stay well. Those with a stronger, more oak-like constitution can take more abuse and get away with it.

Some iridologists like to make another comparison that uses cloth as the illustration. They often compare silk with burlap.

Silk is a very fine weave, soft yet strong, with a high density to its fibers. Burlap is coarse, with a loose weave; it is less dense in its structure. With both the wood and cloth comparisons, the examples used are more or less at the extremes. There are many gradations in between. So it is with body constitution. Overall, a person may have a very strong constitution, a silk or oak type, so to speak, yet within this constitutionally strong body may lurk certain areas of relative weakness, portions that are more like pine or burlap. In fact, this is the norm.

Overall constitution is not representative of each and every area seen in the iris but is a general, or average, assessment of the inherent tissue integrity and strength. To see the difference, merely observe a number of people and note the varying density, or compactness, of their iris fibers. Note, too, that they have areas (sometimes quite a few) where the fibers seem to separate or are just not so densely packed. Notice that these areas usually appear darker than the surrounding portions, where the constitutional integrity of the tissues is stronger.

Observing your constitution, you can see what your parents gave you from a genetic standpoint. This includes the impact of the environment. If your parents were drug addicts and brought down their health, you may have inherited some of the consequences of their indiscretions. Constitution is what you inherently start with in life—your physical dowry. You will have this inherent pattern all your life. Just as certain American Indians weave the history of their tribal family into the designs of their rugs, so you have woven the genetically determined pattern of your inheritance into the warp and woof of the "fabric" of your iris. In this sense, everyone is a man of the cloth, so to speak.

From the starting point of your inheritance, you can develop changes in your iris through exposure to toxic elements in the environment. Air, water, foods, sprays, smoke, drinks, and your adopted lifestyle are all factors that can impose changes over and above your constitutional pattern. A particular way of life determines colorations, inflammations, deposits, and changes—either beneficial or detrimental—as you manage your life. Whatever changes you impose through your living, however, you must remember that you can never change your basic constitutional pattern as visualized in your iris. Understanding your constitution, then, is really your first step in analyzing the structure you inherited. (For an example of an iris with a good constitution, an iris with a poor constitution, and an iris with an average constitution, see Figure 3.3.) *Iridology is primarily a constitutional analysis, whether of the inherent strength or weakness of a particular organ or of the entire body in general. Iridology is the only science that can discern your inherent constitutional strengths and weaknesses—even four generations back.*

Rating Constitution

It is common for iridologists to rate constitution on a scale of one to ten, with one being theoretically perfect and ten being extremely weak. (See Figure 3.1.) Most people fall between three and seven. After you observe a good number of irides, you will be able to judge immediately what number to assign to a particular constitution. Exactness is not necessary in this endeavor. It is not terribly significant if one observer judges a constitution to be a five while another thinks the constitution is a six. One number value one way or the other is not going to matter much. Of course, if you assigned a value of five to an iris that was in actuality closer to an eight, you would be missing the mark significantly and would need more practice.

Look at as many irides as you can. The more you examine, the more accurate you will learn to be. But while rating constitution, remember that it is a gift, an inheritance, and we cannot basically change it. We're stuck with it. It has been said that you cannot make a silk purse out of a sow's ear. We are given a bolt of material—be it silk, cotton, or burlap, so to speak—and we must do with it the best we can. We are all married to our physical body for better or for worse; till death do us part, as they say. We may envy someone else's body, but for better or for worse, we must live with the one we have.

We must affirm that all of God's creation is beautiful. It is by way of iridology that we can come to better see this beauty, in others as well as in ourselves. Knowing our inherent strengths and weaknesses can help us to care for them, to order our lives in such a way that we can capitalize on our strengths while lending a helping hand to our weaknesses. As previously men-

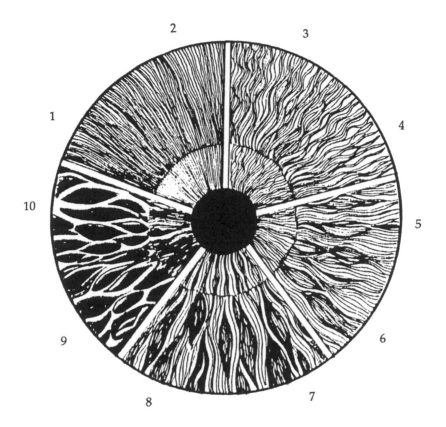

Figure 3.1. Constitution, or fiber quality, is rated on a scale of one to ten. Many iridologists use fabrics as an example when explaining this: silk, with its very fine weave, would be a one; burlap, with its very loose weave, would be a ten. Using woods as an illustration, tight-grained oak would be a one, while loose-grained pine would be a ten. In rating the constitution of an iris, one is theoretically perfect and ten is extremely weak. Most irides fall between three and seven.

tioned, it is a great temptation to assume that constitutional strength is better than weakness. After all, why wouldn't it be better to be strong than to be weak? What possible advantage can there be in weakness? To answer these questions, we must first realize that "better" and "worse" are value judgements not unlike "beautiful" and "ugly." What is better to one person may not be appreciated as such by another.

Weakness displayed in an iris is frequently found in a beautiful person, perhaps a person possessing great strength of character and sensitivity of spirit. Many people with a very strong constitution tend to engage in practices that are detrimental and would bring down the health of someone with lesser inherent strength. They may smoke or drink heavily, or engage in other types of abuse that they can get away with because of their inherent strength. Those with less strength, having relatively weaker constitutions, may find out early in life that they cannot abuse themselves. They may find from experience that they can't take it. Therefore, they must give high consideration to their weaknesses in order to remain symptom-free. Perhaps because of this, they may develop a different outlook on life, becoming more sensitive to the fragilities and needs of others. These people may exhibit more graciousness in adversity and be more attuned to the higher and finer things in life. Who is to say that even though they need to take better care of themselves to stay well, they have received the short end of the stick? Are they necessarily worse off than people with a stronger physical constitution? From my own observations, I conclude that they frequently are not.

Always remember that constitution is not everything in life. It has little, if anything, to do directly with the quality of life. As with the wood in a piece of furniture, constitution does not necessarily play a role in longevity, as long as the individual with the weak constitution exercises due care.

The art of iris analysis requires practice and patience to achieve consistency and a high measure of accuracy. I sometimes refer to the iris as an "instrument of a million strings." I do so because of its numerous fibers. You are now learning to play this incredibly complex and beautiful instrument. But don't think that this skill is developed overnight. There is no substitute for practice.

OPEN AND CLOSED LESIONS

Since you now understand that constitution is a function of the density of iris fibers, we need to go a little further to recognize and classify the various iris signs. An inherent weakness revealed by the iris is nothing more than a limited area with a poorer constitution than its neighboring areas. It's that simple. However, these areas of inherent weakness can take various forms. I will now discuss some of the more common ones.

One of the most common forms an inherent weakness can adopt is known as the "open lesion." Don't let the word "lesion" throw you. Medical people use this word as a sort of catchall for almost any observed physical abnormality. In itself, the word is rather nondescript and is thus usually preceded by one or more adjectives. "Open" is the adjective here, with "open lesion" merely describing a physical shape.

As already mentioned, a lesion often manifests as an area within the fiber structure of the iris, displaying fewer fibers than the regions immediately surrounding it. Therefore, most structural lesions are an area of inherent weakness. A so-called "open lesion" is open at one end, instead of being totally circumscribed. It resembles a corral with a large gate flung open. Thus, open lesions usually resemble a V-shape or a U-shape. In the iris, the open portion of the lesion almost always faces the periphery. Note the example in Figure 3.4. In your analyses, be on the lookout for open lesions.

As you may expect, the other major type of lesion commonly seen in the iris is the closed lesion. (See Figure 3.4 again.) A closed lesion is circumscribed; its border is not broken. It is frequently almond-shaped, although sometimes it is more elongated or spindle-shaped. Other closed lesions appear loop-like and are more apt to be present in weak constitutions, where they are sometimes numerous.

A lesion displaying very white iris fibers is indicating an acute, hyperactive condition. Dark or grey iris lesions correspond with a chronic condition. Black-appearing lesions suggest advanced tissue degeneration. These shadings each represent a different level of tissue integrity. Usually, a lesion is darker than its surrounding, more constitutionally stronger regions. However, one single lesion may contain a dark area as well as some very white fibers. This, of course, indicates an irritation, or acute inflammation, right alongside a chronic condition. This is something to keep in mind when examining a lesion. Lesions need not be homogenous within their borders. There is no reason an area of inflammation cannot exist right next to an area of degeneration, with both inside the same inherent weakness. Be on the lookout for this situation when you see either a closed or open lesion.

Some open lesions have a very distinct border, the same as closed lesions do. Others do not. Often, an open lesion may be manifest simply as an area of diminished fiber density, with little or no discrete border. Of course, if chronic and toxic, the region will appear dark. If not darker than the surrounding iris fibers, it will merely be an inherent weakness with a lower fiber density and not in a chronic or degenerative condition.

Try to observe as many irides as possible and look for different examples of both open and closed lesions so that you can learn how to easily differentiate between them. Remember, open lesions are less distinct because they sometimes do not have neatly circumscribed borders. In addition, they are nearly always open at the end toward the periphery of the iris. Closed lesions may be elongated, almond-shaped, round, or irregular, but have more easily defined, circumscribed borders.

Now that we have a working knowledge of constitution— what it is, how to rate it, and what signs to look for—let's move on to an examination of a major landmark in the iris.

THE AUTONOMIC NERVE WREATH

A major iris landmark is a structure called the "autonomic nerve wreath." (See Figure 3.5.) This wreath is sometimes called the "iris frill." Look for it about one-third of the way out from the pupil. On the iris chart, it is labelled "autonomic nervous system."

The autonomic nerve wreath resembles a somewhat jagged or scalloped ring. The color and structure of the iris will appear somewhat different inside this ring than in the rest of the iris. The color is usually significantly darker inside the nerve wreath, and the fiber structure inside it is looser, or coarser, in texture. The wreath itself usually appears somewhat raised, like the ridge of a mountain chain, if you can picture the iris as the topographical map that it truly is.

If you are thinking that the constitution of the area inside the wreath is somewhat inherently weaker than that of the area outside the wreath, you are right on track. I have yet to see a structure within the wreath that is as constitutionally strong as the average structure outside the wreath. This observation is very important and I will have more to say about it later.

The wreath itself represents the autonomic nervous system. Don't let the word "autonomic" scare you. The autonomic system is comprised of two subsystems that tend to offset each other in their functioning, much like the two arms of a balanced scale. It is healthy and normal for these two systems to be in balance. The two systems are the sympathetic nervous system and the parasympathetic nervous system. Together, they are considered a single entity, namely the autonomic nervous system. Iridologists, when referring to the autonomic nerve wreath in the iris, often drop the word "autonomic" and just say "the nerve wreath," or even more simply, "the wreath." Whatever you choose to call it, it is a major landmark that you cannot neglect.

Take some time now to see if you can locate the nerve wreath. The more irides you look at, the more accurate you will become. Remember, the wreath is seldom as stylized as it appears on the iris chart. Also, it is not always located at the classic one-third distance from the edge of the pupil to the iris periphery. Sometimes it is quite close to the pupil, while other times it is situated much further out. In most cases, it is quite scalloped and uneven. Sometimes it appears rather jagged, dipping in close to the pupil in one area and then jutting out again in another. In some irides, it is more difficult to see, but with experience, you will see it clearly nearly every time. Take note of its shape in every iris you examine and be aware that each wreath is as unique to a person as his fingerprint.

IRIS SIGNS ON THE NERVE WREATH

There are several iris signs visualized on the autonomic nerve wreath. When visualized, they manifest as a disturbance in the normal character of the wreath at their iris-chart location. They concern the heart, thymus gland, which is not depicted on some iris charts, and solar plexus, which is labelled "sol. pl." on the chart. Let's consider the heart first.

It is important to realize that not *all* heart problems reveal themselves as a wreath disturbance. The heart is a muscle, but it is a special muscle, composed of unique tissue. It is also different because it is highly innervated, that is, served by a large and complex bundle of nerves. These nerves help control its pulses. Some types of heart disturbances are associated with problems in the nerve supply. Other conditions are not related to the nerve supply at all. Two examples of the latter type are muscular problems and vascular obstructive problems. Usually, vascular obstructive problems are the ones associated with the common angina pain and heart attack we have become so familiar with. These are not heart problems as much as they are vascular problems that can have a chronic, or sometimes sudden, effect on an otherwise healthy heart.

I will comment on circulatory problems later. First, I want to separate the heart conditions associated with nerve function from those linked to vascular conditions because cardiovascular conditions do not generally reveal themselves in the heart area on the iris chart. In addition, neither do they manifest as a disturbance of the autonomic nerve wreath, as do inherited weaknesses associated with nerve supply to the heart. Inherited heart weaknesses involving nerve supply manifest as a separation of the nerve wreath in the heart area. Please notice on the iris chart that the heart and the solar plexus do not merely border the nerve wreath but are actually an integral part of it.

The iris sign to look for concerning an inherited heart weakness involving the nerve supply to this vital organ is a separation of the autonomic nerve wreath with a joining again in the heart area of the iris chart. This produces a diamond-shaped or trapezoidal-shaped lesion where the wreath separation occurs. It is like a river splitting into two equal-sized streams that unite again after forming a diamond-shaped island in midstream. As with other lesions, you can check this island for an acute, chronic, or degenerative appearance. However, you must be extremely cautious not to mistake a dark bowel pocket opposite the heart area for a chronic or degenerative heart lesion. Even the experienced iridologist sometimes has trouble distinguishing between a bowel pocket and a heart lesion.

It is wise to refrain from commenting on a possible heart condition observed in the iris. You could needlessly upset a person, causing him a great deal of fear and anguish. This is a matter that is best left to a health professional.

The second sign to look for on the nerve wreath concerns the thymus gland. The thymus gland is not depicted on some early Jensen iris charts. When it is illustrated, however, it is found in the left iris, immediately below the heart area. I will say more about the thymus later, in the section on glands. The important thing to notice now is that like the heart, the thymus is positioned directly on the autonomic nerve wreath. And like the heart, signs of problems affecting this gland are wreath disturbances such as abnormal thickening, thinning, and breaking in the wreath. As you will learn later, a range of white to black near the wreath at this gland location can also be significant.

The solar plexus is the third anatomical entity located on the nerve wreath. Note its location in the left iris, not far below the heart and thymus,. The solar plexus is also known as the "celiac plexus." There is much metaphysical lore surrounding the functions of this nerve plexus. A plexus, however, is nothing more than a collection of, and distribution point for, numerous nerve bundles. It's like an electrical substation, where many electrical lines come in from various points, interconnect, and then move out again to other locations.

The solar plexus is the largest of the body's three great autonomic nerve plexuses. Nerves from the solar plexus serve the liver, gall bladder, abdominal arteries, tissues of the bowel as far down as the rectum, stomach, diaphragm, spleen, kidneys, adrenal glands, ovaries, and testes. An inherent weakness in the autonomic nerve wreath at the location of the solar plexus indicates a weak nerve supply in, or to, this plexus. Thus, the organs served by the plexus are probably suffering from a diminished, or aberrant, nerve supply.

As you examine an iris, look for an abnormally thin or thick section on the autonomic nerve wreath at the three locations mentioned: heart, thymus, and solar plexus. If the wreath appears thick, white, and elevated, it indicates an acute condition with an overactivity of nerve energy. If thin and thready, it indicates a weakened nerve flow. If the wreath shows a trapezoid-shaped split at the heart area, note the degree of whiteness or darkness. This, as you shall further see, indicates the degree of acuteness or chronicity.

Now that you have seen some signs *on* the wreath, it's time to consider some signs *inside* the wreath.

IRIS SIGNS INSIDE THE NERVE WREATH

Inside the autonomic nerve wreath are several more iris signs. Two of the areas involved overlap each other. A third area is not depicted. Look at the iris chart, at the area inside the nerve wreath. Can you see which two areas might overlap each other? Proceeding outward from the pupil, they are the circular stomach area and the interrupted, ring-like intestinal area. The intestinal area is bordered inwardly by the pupilary margin and outwardly by the scalloped autonomic nerve wreath. Please note that *on the chart*, the areas depicting the intestines and stomach do not overlap; they appear separate and distinct. This, however, is for illustrative purposes only. In practice, these two areas do overlap. I will discuss the intestinal area first.

In practice, as indicated on the chart, the intestinal area is always bordered outwardly by the autonomic nerve wreath. So you can see that a fairly large area, from the pupil edge to the wreath and circumscribing the pupil, represents the intestines, or bowel. The iris signs associated with the intestinal area are a general overall darkness and a poorer constitution inside the wreath than outside. You will always be able to define the approximate intestinal area by these two signs, even if the wreath cannot be visualized well. The importance of the intestinal area and its relative darkness will soon be seen.

A significant and variable portion of the intestinal area also represents the stomach. It helps to think of the stomach ring as resembling a photographic double exposure. The stomach ring, when visualized, overlays the bowel area, creating the effect of a double-exposed picture. The stomach visualized as part of the intestine has its anatomical correlation to the body: since the stomach is but a distended pouch in the digestive tract and not a separate, detached organ apart from the bowel, it is visualized, when manifest, as overlaying the bowel area.

When the stomach is properly functioning, the stomach sign is not visualized in the iris as distinct from the intestines. In other words, *no iris sign is seen for the stomach when the stomach is functioning well.* Instead, when the stomach is functioning properly, the sign resembles a clear, transparent overlay on the intestinal area between the wreath and the pupil. The stomach sign does make an appearance, however, if the stomach's function, or tissue integrity, is other than normal—if it is overactive or underactive. When manifest, the sign appears as a perfectly circumscribed ring of discoloration. (See Figure 3.6.) It always appears perfectly round and has a smooth circumference. It may concentrically overlay either a portion of the intestinal area inside the wreath or the entire area inside the wreath, and in some instances, it may extend out beyond the wreath for a short distance. Remember that even when it is seen, it is not visualized in the iris as a *structure,* but only as a slight-to-moderate variant in color or hue. It is when the wreath is very close to the pupil that the stomach ring may appear to extend out beyond the borders of the wreath.

Looking again at the iris chart, please note the labels "pylorus" and "cardia" within the stomach area. The pylorus is the little valve connecting the stomach to the duodenum, which is labelled "duo" on the chart. The duodenum is an area where ulcers commonly occur. "Cardia" refers to the area where the stomach connects to the esophagus. "Kardia," as you may know, is the Greek word meaning "heart." The curvature of the stomach near the esophageal entrance is somewhat heart-shaped, thus suggesting the terminology.

As you carry out your observations, you won't find the stomach ring present in every iris, but you will find it in quite a few. Take a moment to look for it. Depending on its hue, it indicates either too much or too little hydrochloric acid in the stomach. It is much more common for the stomach to be under-acidic than over-acidic. Under-acidity and over-acidity correspond directly with overactivity and underactivity of the stomach tissues, not of the stomach contents. Improper amounts of

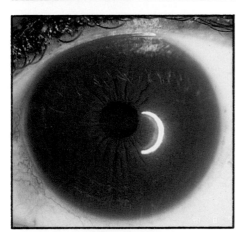

Blue

Brown

Mixed

Figure 3.2. Irides are either basically blue (top photo), basically brown (middle photo), or mixed (bottom photo).

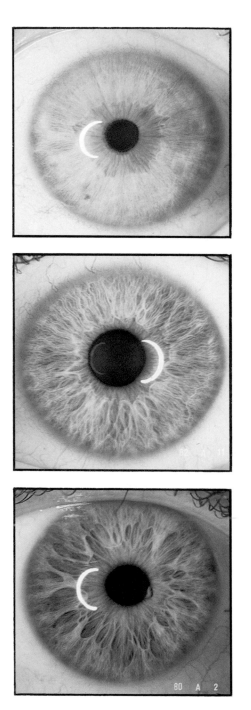

Good

Average

Poor

Figure 3.3. Iridologists classify constitution on a scale of 1 to 10, with good (top photo) falling between 1 and 3; average (middle photo), between 4 and 7; and poor (bottom photo), between 8 and 10.

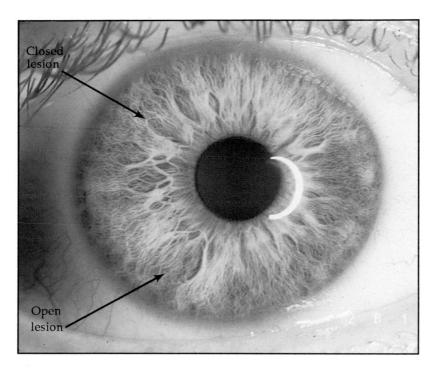

Open lesion and closed lesion

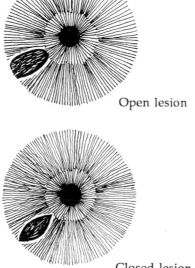

Open lesion

Closed lesion

Figure 3.4. The open lesion resembles a corral with the gate flung open. It is usually V-shaped or U-shaped. The closed lesion has a perfectly circumscribed border. It is usually almond-shaped but sometimes elongated, spindle-shaped, or loop-like.

Plate 4   *Visions of Health*

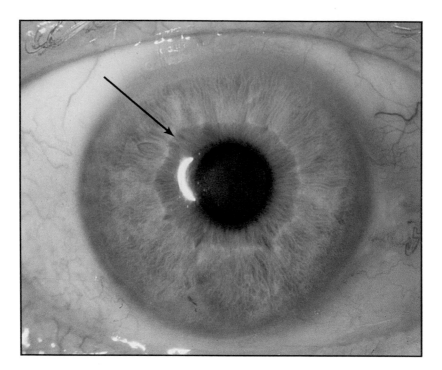

Autonomic nerve wreath

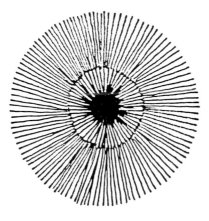

Figure 3.5. The autonomic nerve wreath is the jagged or scalloped ring about one-third of the way out from the pupil. It represents the autonomic nervous system.

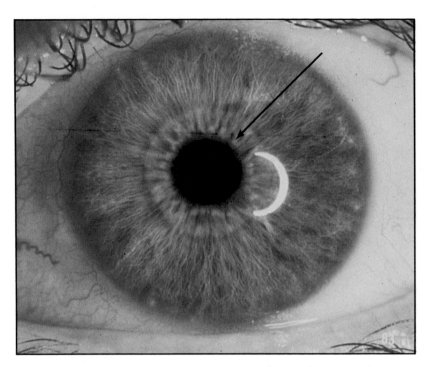

Overactive stomach

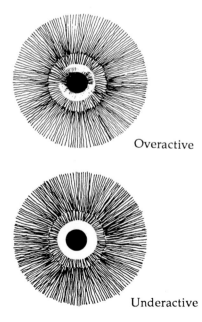

Overactive

Underactive

Figure 3.6. The stomach sign, when visible, is a perfectly circumscribed ring of discoloration. When light-colored, it indicates the stomach is overactive, or has too much acid. When dark, it shows the stomach is underactive. It is transparent when the stomach is fine. Here, it is indicating overactivity.

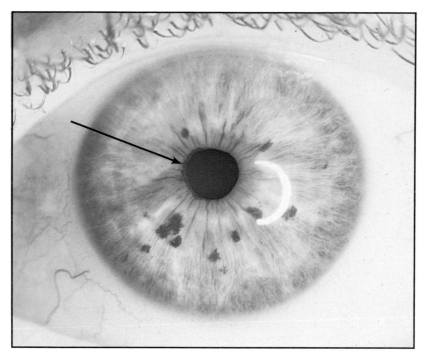

Absorption ring

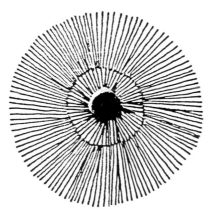

Figure 3.7. When an absorption ring is present, it means that nutrient absorption from the small intestine is compromised. Look for a reddish-brown or burnt-umber edge around the pupil.

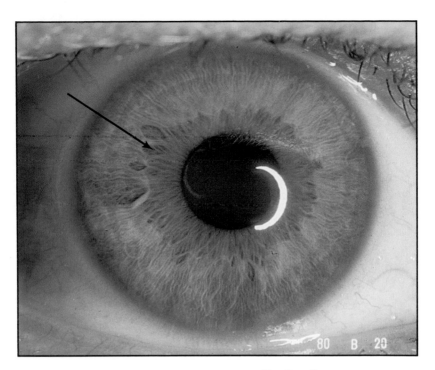

Healing lines

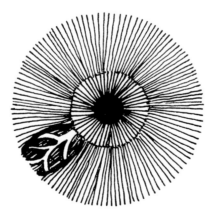

Figure 3.8. Healing lines indicate that old, damaged tissue is being replaced with new, healthy tissue. Visualizing them is the goal of the iridologist.

Plate 8   *Visions of Health*

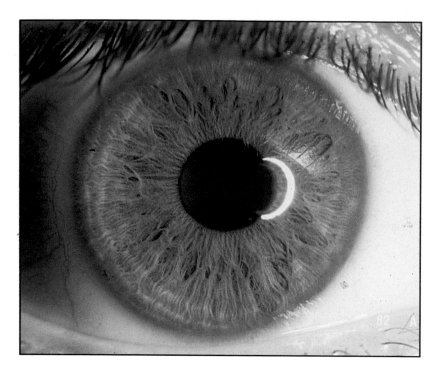

Miasm

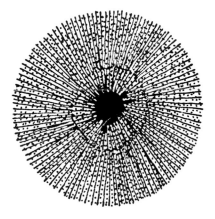

Figure 3.9. A miasmic iris is also called a "dishwater eye" because of its murky, lackluster color. The effect is often from some type of body pollution, such as a medication or environmental toxin.

stomach acid are associated with digestive dysfunction. Both too much and too little are connected with dysfunction and may also be associated with disease. (For an explanation of how overactivity and underactivity are determined, please see "The Stomach Ring," on page 52.)

The stomach ring is one of the signs that may not be easily visualized by the beginner. It is especially difficult to find in dark brown irides. As with most of the other iris signs, it is better to begin by examining light colored eyes. When you can discern the sign well in light eyes, go on to darker eyes. Compare your findings with Figure 3.6.

There are times when the stomach sign is visible but does not necessarily indicate altered function. This is a relatively rare occurrence that is better left for a more in-depth study of iridology. It takes an expert with a lot of experience to discern the presence of a stomach ring in some irides. As in most endeavors, practice makes better. There is no perfection in health care, which is why doctors are always practicing.

The third "area" inside the autonomic nerve wreath is not depicted on the chart. There is good reason for this. Known as the "absorption ring," it is like the stomach ring, an indicator of function only. It is not an anatomical structure. And like the stomach ring, it indicates proper and normal function by its absence. Its not being visualized indicates good nutrient absorption from the small intestine.

When the absorption ring is present, it is visualized just around the inside of the pupilary margin (see Figure 3.7). When looking at an iris, look for a reddish-brown or burnt-umber-colored edge, called the "pupilary ruff," which signals a degree of absorptive dysfunction. The wider the ring is, the greater is the degree of dysfunction. Take a moment to see if you can find an iris showing an absorption ring. The appearance of a slight ring is not so rare as to be unusual. I think few people have as good absorption as they should have.

These, then, are the basic things to look for in an iris: first, color; next, constitution; and then, signs around the autonomic nerve wreath. These alone will give you a wealth of information about the body behind the eyes. Why? That's in Chapter 4.

The Stomach Ring

The stomach ring, when visualized, is an indicator of the tissue integrity of the stomach wall. In practice, this tissue integrity is directly related to the amount of acid produced by the stomach. Stomach acid is needed to protect the digestive tract from harmful organisms and to acidify stomach contents in preparation for their entrance into the small intestine. The stomach wall itself normally has high concentrations of sodium, an alkaline mineral, which serves to protect the stomach lining from the erosive effect of the acid. Thus, a balance is maintained between the acid contents and the alkaline wall.

As we enter our middle years, our glandular output begins to slow down. The secretion of stomach acid also slows. In addition, if we do not maintain a sufficient intake of organic sodium, the stomach wall may become depleted of adequate sodium stores. This shortage can be compounded by the slowing down of other glands, especially the thyroid.

A significant loss of sodium in the stomach wall can result in the formation of an ulcer as the acid irritates the stomach or duodenal lining. It's important to note here that worries and fears tend to burn out sodium reserves and upset digestive processes and glandular balance. There is truth in the old adage, "You don't get ulcers from what you eat. You get them from what's eating you." Worry, fear, and stress cause the body to secrete strong and noxious acids that literally poison and irritate all the cells and can drive the whole system to become so over-acidic that the best diet cannot compensate.

With all this in mind, we are now ready to take a closer look at the stomach ring. This is an advanced topic; properly analyzing a stomach ring takes much practice to perfect. Not every stomach ring you visualize will indicate overactivity or underactivity to the degree you initially conclude. To determine the activity of stomach tissue, you should compare the hue of the visualized ring with the hue of the fibers outside the nerve wreath that represent the best constitution in the iris. We can make a generalization here and say that if the stomach ring is darker than these fibers, it represents an underactive stomach. If lighter, it represents an overactive stomach. That's rather straightforward, even if it is not as easy as it sounds. The observation, however, is complicated by the need to also take into consideration the systemic acid level, as represented by the overall whiteness of the iris fibers. If the fibers are in general whiter than they should be, the stomach ring by comparison will appear darker and you might think that it is more underactive than it really is.

You can see, therefore, that overactivity or underactivity of the stomach is determined by comparing hues that are sometimes very difficult to properly compare. In addition, the comparison may be made even more difficult by the degree of systemic acidity, revealed by the whiteness of the iris fibers, and it may also be hampered by the relative darkness of the intestinal tract, which the stomach ring overlays. Because of the difficulty presented by the number of factors involved and the relativity of each one to the others, the stomach ring can frequently present a challenge to even the most experienced iridologist. The computerized analysis of the iris in the future may better deal with the complexities of the stomach ring.

4.

Focus on How and Why

T he eye, with its iris, is a direct outgrowth of the brain. The eye is the only brain tissue that can be directly seen without surgical intervention. This is very important. When a doctor uses an ophthalmoscope to peer through the pupil and view the retina, he is actually looking at a part of the brain.

Not many days after the gleam in your father's eye was shared with your mother, the cells that were to become your eyes began to bud out from your brain, not unlike the new buds on a tree. In so doing, they trailed behind them a kind of neurological umbilical cord, their communication link to the parental brain centers. This connecting link evolved in time into the optic nerve.

The optic nerve, although referred to in the singular, is in actuality a nerve bundle, comprised of hundreds of thousands of individual nerve fibers. It is much like a large cable supporting a suspension bridge. It is composed of numerous smaller units, each of which is made up of even smaller units, until there are a nearly countless number of tiny, individual strands. Some of the fibers in the optic nerve terminate in the iris. Thus, there is a nerve pathway over which messages travel back and forth between the brain and the iris.

The brain is the CPU (computer talk for "central processing unit") of the entire organism. It knows what is going on in all parts of the body. It then relays the information easily to the iris using the optic nerve as its path. Can you visualize the pathway over which information is conveyed from your little toe, via the brain, to your iris? It is very much like the system that causes one end of a cat to yell when you step on its other end!

When an iridologist looks into an eye, he is not looking at a diseased eye that will be treated as such. He is looking at a monitor screen, a surface that is displaying the tissue integrity in other parts of the body. Information about the condition of these remote tissues is routed first to the brain, via spinal-cord pathways, and then to the eye, for display on the iris "video terminal." The iris is indicating the functional ability and inherent structural makeup of the distant tissues. It is telling the iridologist the relative amount of toxic settlement in those tissues and their chemical nutritional deficiency. No other form of analysis or diagnosis can discern all these things and be completely noninvasive.

To understand what is showing up in the iris, you will need to learn iridology's language and philosophy. You will need these tools to understand manifestations that cannot be explained by the terminology, philosophy, and current understanding of orthodox medicine. In this chapter, I will continue to introduce you to these tools, plus I will explain how and why iridology works.

A SPECIAL KIND OF REFLEXOLOGY

Iridology is based upon the principles of reflexology. Reflexes are a well-known and accepted biological and physiological phenomenon. What schoolboy doesn't know that a thumbtack carefully placed on a chair provokes an immediate, and usually colorful, exclamatory response? Doctors learn that a strike just below the knee with a little rubber percussion hammer normally elicits an immediate jerk of the leg. This "knee jerk," as it is called, is an important measure of a properly functioning spinal-nerve pathway. It is a simple test of the reflexes. People cannot live without good reflexes. They protect us from injury and even death. Many an accident is averted by quick reflexes. With age, our reflexes become slower. Still, every doctor knows that good reflex response is the mark of an intact and properly functioning nervous system.

By way of illustration, you might think of television as a kind of reflex system. The camera focuses on a subject and transmits a picture of it to a distant receiver. Whatever the camera sees is in turn faithfully reproduced on the television screen. Iridology can be thought of in this way, too. What is seen in the discrete iris fibers is merely an indication of what is taking place in another area of the body. The brain knows all. It is the master of the body. It knows what is going on in every part of the system. Without it, you cannot live. There isn't anything that happens in your body that your brain doesn't know about. It monitors every corner of your biological real estate and continually transmits this information to your irides.

Very little of what the brain knows is brought to consciousness. Most of the activity of the brain is apart from any conscious realization or thought process. For instance, you need not give a single thought to the number of times your heart beats each minute. But your brain knows. You also don't need to think about increasing your breathing rate with more strenuous activity. You don't have to be conscious of that—but your brain is. And as a result, your brain is constantly sending signals to make the adjustments necessary for your survival and well-being. Since the eyes are highly specialized brain tissue, they, too, know what's what in the body. And what they know is revealed in the iris.

Educators tell us that 86 percent of all we learn comes through the eyes. The ears are responsible for only 6 percent, and the remaining senses account for only an additional 7 percent. Scientists tell us that the eyes can see 8 million colors. An estimated 500,000 nerves connect the iris with the brain. Is it any wonder that the iris, the eye tissue, holds so much knowledge? You will be dealing with an unimaginable and wondrous complexity when examining an iris.

Since the nervous system employs a vast distribution of nerve endings to all parts of the body, information is continually relayed to and from the brain. Health-care systems using areas of the body other than the irides have also been developed. The best known systems utilize the hands and feet. Specialists who work in these areas are usually known as reflexologists. The iridologist can be considered a special kind of reflexologist.

Other reflexology systems differ from iridology in that the practitioner must physically touch the client, massaging, manipulating, pressing, or vibrating the involved areas with the fingers or a variety of small hand tools. The reflexologist is guided to some degree by the client's response to his efforts. Thus, a measure of discomfort can sometimes be associated with other reflexology techniques. The important thing to remember is that unlike iridology, nearly all other forms of reflexology depend upon physical contact, rather than being confined to visual observation.

Reflexologists believe that physical stimulation of precise nerve endings on the palms of the hand or soles of the feet causes the brain to relay messages to the corresponding organs of the body. This nerve stimulation enhances the flow of nerve energy and promotes the restoration of balance in the affected areas, as well as eventually reducing pain and discomfort at the stimulation site. Some years ago, a Rochester, New York, nurse named Eunice D. Ingham wrote several books on foot reflexology that helped to promote this form of therapy. In her books, she outlined zones of the body that closely resemble the meridians described in acupuncture. In fact, she referred to the practice of foot reflexology as "zone therapy." Common to all forms of reflexology, including iridology, is the structuring of a chart or map that depicts the location of the zones and organs of the area, be it the feet, hands, irides, or another body part.

Unlike other forms of reflexology, iridology does not necessitate physical contact with the client's body. Neither does it require stimulation of any kind using the fingers or another instrument. The iridologist merely observes. With iridology, you look but don't touch. It is also important to remember that iridology is *non*therapeutic. It does not involve itself directly in therapy or treatment. Instead, it is a form of analysis. Of course, iridologists who are professionals licensed to provide a certain type of health-care service can recommend an appropriate therapeutic regimen utilizing the information gleaned from an iris analysis.

THE IRIS CHART AND HERING'S LAW OF CURE

In Chapter 2, I discussed the iris chart and how its construction is related to body function. This relation to function can be seen best in what is known as Hering's Law of Cure. Although hardly a household name today, Constantine Hering was a nineteenth-century European homeopathic physician of some repute. Through his work as a clinician, he formulated a law of healing that maintains that disease is cured by a reversal process.

The iris chart is constructed according to Hering's Law. Hering's Law states: *All cure starts from within out, from the head down, and in the reverse order as the symptoms appeared.* In other words, as you begin to think, eat, and live in a more healthful way, you experience, in reverse order, all the conditions and symptoms that led to your present unhealthy condition. This reversal continues until you arrive at a state of well-being once again. Doctors who employ nature's ways find Hering's Law of Cure to be confirmed in practice. They also find that any significant departure from nature's ordinations will slow, if not stop, this reversal process.

Hering's Law of Cure also states that healing takes place from within out. If you will again look at the iris chart on page 22–23, you will see in its organization that the pupil is the most central entity. It is the hub. As already mentioned, educators say that about 86 percent of all learning comes by way of the visual sense. They believe that we retain more of what we see than of what we take in through any of our other senses. Seeing is believing, they say.

We should also consider yet another sight that does not depend upon the eyes or, for that matter, on any of the five senses. This sight is *in*sight, as when someone says, "I see what you mean." Both types of sight involve brain activity. It is a fact of life that a person tends to become what is on his mind most often. What we see and hold in our mind's eye is transformed into actuality over time. If sickness, despondent thoughts, and ill health are on your mind, you are likely to find yourself in such condition before long. Conversely, if you concentrate on the pure and wholesome side of life, with feelings of satisfaction and well being, you will more likely move into the future in good physical and mental health.

How do you see yourself? What insights do you have about yourself? How you think of yourself is an important part of your diet of inner thoughts. It is no less real than a diet of food. It's food for thought. Thought is our most inward activity. It is part of what Dr. Hering meant when he said that all healing begins on the inside and moves outward.

Frequently, I point out in my lectures that you have to feel better before you can feel better. By that, I mean that you must feel better in your mind before you can feel better in your body. You feel with your mind first. Joy is felt in the mind, not in the heart. The physical side of life is subservient to, and thus follows, the mental side. Psychologists refer to this as the "psychosomatic" connection, the influence of mind on body; of inner, intangible thought on outward, tangible flesh. As you can see, this is in accordance with Hering's Law, which maintains that healing moves down from the head and out from the inside. This is why the pupil must be at the center of the chart and why all healing moves not only down from the head, but also out from within. What is a pupil anyway but one who takes in, one who learns? We are influenced by what we take in. Take in and learn joy. You were created for joy. You will find that as your mind becomes more joyful and positive, health and healing begin to manifest in your body.

As within, so without, say the sages. In Hering's Law, the truth of the spiritual and mental sides of healing are made congruent with the physical laws of wellness. Don't deny yourself what only you can give yourself. The basic concepts of the iris chart are a spiritual gift to mankind. With the aid of the modern iris chart and Hering's Law, we are privileged to see the central idea of wholism—the body-mind-spirit connection.

Another aspect of Hering's Law is that in order to get well, a person must experience a healing in each damaged organ or system, going in this reverse order from the pupil outward. Doctors always find it difficult to treat a person who has a bad attitude or is depressed. They know from experience that this person will have a very difficult time getting well, no matter what the physical problem may be or which treatments are prescribed. So, you can see right away that all healing must start at the most inward place. This means your insight, your thoughts, your attitude, the way you see things. Your feelings and mental condition correspond to the pupil on the iris chart. If your attitude needs changing, look at things in a different way. Only you can allow yourself to see things differently.

I am a chiropractor, but I can truthfully say that the greatest adjustment is not made in the spine but in the attitude. A greater need exists for attitude adjustment than even for spinal adjustment. In my lectures, I often remark that your attitude is your altitude. It's impossible to have high thoughts while feeling low.

Sometimes we need a new outlook on life. Physical outlook comes through the pupil, but mental outlook comes from the mind. You might call it "inlook." You may need to take stock of yourself, make an inventory. People get new ideas this way. People who go within themselves for their new ideas are known as "*in*ventors." There are also people who are always blowing off. They have the same time-worn litany of complaints and nothing new or happy to talk about. Instead of changing inwardly, they vent all their problems outwardly to whomever will listen. It's best to stay away from these people.

Our spiritual outlook is nurtured from a new uplook. No one ever reached for the stars with his eyes downcast. When things are looking up in life, it's usually because you are feeling good about yourself. A person is more than the sum of his physical parts. This is the philosophy hidden in Hering's Law.

Let me tell you how healing takes place according to Hering's Law. Healing is like a pebble dropped into still water. On the iris chart, it begins at the pupil and moves in ever-widening concentric circles toward the periphery. We already discussed the mental side of life and the importance of what we take in through the pupil. Now let's move outward. After the pupil come the stomach and bowel. You cannot have good digestion without a good stomach, or a good heart without a good bowel and good digestion. Note again that the stomach and digestive tract surround the pupil and that nearly all the other organs and areas take off radially from the digestive tract.

All healing moves from within out. *It's impossible for most things to work properly without a well-functioning digestive system.* As proof, statistics show that more hospital admissions are associated with digestive complaints than with anything else. Working with the chart, going in reverse order, we can affirm that most digestive troubles are associated with emotional problems, fears, stresses, phobias, mental problems, and sour human relationships.

As a chiropractor, I often have to counsel patients about their pain in the neck. I have also listened to them tell me about a pain in the neck where they work. It may be their boss. It may be a fellow employee. Sometimes the problem is at home, with a wife, husband, or children. As a doctor, I know that they cannot get rid of their pain in the neck until they make peace with themselves. I have often said in my lectures that nothing can harm you unless you give it your consent. Make sure you don't let things get to you. Never forget that you're the only one who has control over this. No one else can keep things from bothering you. You must deal with these problems from within.

The dermatologist is one of the busiest doctors in town. Let's see if we can figure out why. Look at where the skin is depicted on the iris chart. It is the outermost part of the body and is represented in zone 7, the periphery of the chart. If all healing moves from the inside out, then according to the chart, the skin is the last organ to be affected. If you suppose that almost anything amiss in the body can manifest itself as a skin condition, you're thinking according to Hering's Law. Every doctor has seen an emotional stress produce hives in a matter of minutes. Bowel problems, liver conditions, and other abnormalities can also affect the skin. It serves little good or lasting purpose to apply lotions and cremes to the skin while neglecting to consider the more inward causes. Now you know why the dermatologist is the busiest doctor in town.

My desire is that you see the validity of Hering's Law and its intimate association with iris-chart construction. All healing takes place from within out. You have seen that the iris chart is wonderfully constructed according to Hering's Law and that the chart's form relates to physical function. Hering's Law of Cure and the chart confirm each other's validity.

All iris charts were developed empirically, through years of careful clinical observation. What is depicted on them has been experienced by iridologists time and time again. Of course, this does not make any chart perfect. No responsible iridologist would ever suggest that such is the case. But all iris charts, by whomever constructed, display a marked similarity to one another. Some are nearly identical, revealing only minor differences. And all the iris charts that I have seen are in keeping with Hering's Law.

HERING'S LAW IN ACTION

Hering's Law in action is known as the "reversal process." The reversal process takes place when a person who has been on a sick, chronic, downhill path decides to stop, turn around, and reverse his direction. I already indicated that this first step is always a mental step, a decision. It's taking your health and life into your own hands, making a private decision, and going your own way. It is not leaving it all to the doctor, patronizing the local pharmacist, and going along in the same old habits that brought on the trouble in the first place. No, it is an attitude adjustment, followed with new habits, a casting off of the old and putting on of the new. It is a retracing process, a path that leads to restored health. It is the rebuilding of tissue integrity. The reversal process, according to Hering's Law, is the only way to true health and wholeness. Other methods may provide symptom relief, but relief without correction leads only to continued loss of tissue integrity and a more chronic or degenerative condition.

Wise men say that the only constant in life is change. You should particularly remember this in regard to health. We are either building or destroying our health at any given moment. The health, or integrity, of every cell in our body is in constant flux. Not to choose the way that builds health is to default and suffer the consequences of degeneration. Millions of new cells are created each day in the body as old ones die off. Will the new ones have a greater integrity or lesser integrity than the previous ones? Will they serve their purpose well? In time, will the iris indicate a diminished tissue integrity or one that is stronger and more vibrant? The choice is ours.

The goal of iridology is to visualize tissue changes in the iris that are indications of an improved tissue integrity. (See Figure 4.1. See also Figure 3.8 in Chapter 3.) This is true healing. Replacing old tissue with new, healthy cells is, in reality, the only healing worthy of the name. I do not mean mere symptom relief or remedy. I am outlining a process of reconstruction, a

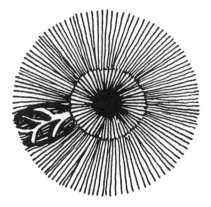

Figure 4.1. Healing lines
show that healing is tak-
ing place. For a photo-
graph, see Figure 3.9.

remodeling job, where new materials are inserted in place of the
old. This is not suppression. No cover-up job here! This is a
grassroots project, a new-from-the-inside-out endeavor.

Disease and poor health are more often made than born.
People choose by default to trek down the path of ill health, a
path that leads to ever-more chronic disease. This path is broad
and easy, a path of ignorance, ease, foolishness, and neglect.
Some people have a wrong diet, some have wrong thinking,
others have a wrong job, and perhaps others even have the
wrong marriage partner. Nowhere more than in health do two
wrongs fail to make a right. Each wrong pushes us a little
further down the path to destruction, with its corresponding
loss of tissue integrity. As we take more drugs and nostrums to
relieve the symptoms, we travel further down the path. We have
come a very long way down the path and are very near the end
when the doctor admits that there is nothing more he can do.
"You just have to learn to live with it," he says. This is the path
of suppression, the way of drugs, remedies, and nostrums
taken for relief. In my lectures, I tell people that we live in a
relief society. We've been on relief for too long. Learning to live
with chronic disease while taking drugs for the partial and
temporary relief of symptoms is the reward for bad living habits
and short-cut remedies.

Most people do not do the things that bring correction.

Instead, they go along in their old ways. It's business as usual. They do not replace old thoughts with new thoughts or old tissue with new, improved tissue, but merely use drugs to alleviate their symptoms. Thus, they continue to struggle along in the same established patterns and old habits, moving down the broad and easy road to ever-greater chronicity and degeneration. In order to reverse the downward spiral toward degeneration and ill health, we must first stop the health-destroying habits that have become part and parcel of our lifestyle. Iris analysis demonstrates that the only genuine way back to health is to reverse our path. Why not go all out for a healthy body? Why not stop the self-destructive ways of living and do an about-face? How about giving up bad habits and installing healthful ones in their place? Why not learn to be our body's best friend, instead of our own worst enemy?

A popular expression says that the body is a garden and the mind is its caretaker. The condition of our garden depends greatly upon the habits of its caretaker. Habits—good and bad—tend to be enduring. I would like to tell you about habits. Do you know why it's so difficult to break a habit? A habit is an H-A-B-I-T. If you take away the H, you have A-BIT. If you take away the A, you still have a BIT. Take away the B and you still have IT. Do you see why a habit is so hard to break? To chisel away at a bad habit seldom works. You must give it up cold turkey and be done with it. Just stop. Reaffirm who is in control and assert your higher self. Habits being what they are, you really need to be very careful to establish the kind of habits that will serve you well in life and not lead you down the wrong path. If you don't like where you live, get out. The average person just goes through life without making too many changes. Your first job on the road to better health is to change your thinking away from the average. To visualize the healing process in the iris, you must find out what constitutes better living and adopt those better ways. Drop the old and take up the new. For most people, this means major changes in their life.

You should not continue in life as an average person because the average person is not as well as he should be. The average person lives with a chronic or degenerative condition. Sometimes, he is aware of the condition and is content to nurse it along if the inconvenience is not too great. Other times, he is totally unaware of the chronic condition, which, without a change in habits, continues to progress toward the degenerative. Remember, the average is always significantly lower than the best. The average person may not even realize in what a chronic state of health he is. When he is aware, he doesn't know how to care for himself properly. He doesn't know how to employ nature to assist him with restoring his health. You must be above average if you want to get well and stay well. You must learn more than the average person learns, do differently than the average person does. The average person has developed many bad health habits. You cannot build a new structure while continuing the unhealthy habits of the average person. Figures show that eight of every ten people who say they feel well are found, when examined, to have a chronic disease.

Every person utilizing iris analysis looks for iris signs indicating that new structure is developing in the various organs of the body. They look for signs of healing, of the raising of tissue integrity. Finding these signs is the ultimate goal of iris analysis. The iris indicates if the person has traded his bad habits for better ones. It tells what path the person has been following lately. It doesn't take too long to see whether or not a person has risen above the average. You can see these special iris signs for yourself when you take a look at your own irides or those of a friend.

DISEASE AS OVERACTIVITY OR UNDERACTIVITY

Disease has been called "normal function gone wrong." It is function altered at the cellular level. When we have a *dis*ease or don't feel well, we have something out of balance. We are not as we were ordained to be. Our normal function has been altered. Something is off center.

D. D. Palmer, the nineteenth-century father of chiropractic, the second largest healing profession in the United States, claimed that abnormality in bodily function is directly related to overactivity or underactivity of the nerve supply to body tissues. He claimed that this, in turn, caused the tissues to become functionally overactive or underactive. He said that too much or too little nerve supply to tissues led, in time, directly to disease. Although this idea was put forth by the founder of modern chiropractic shortly after the turn of this century, it is by no means limited to the practice of chiropractic. Palmer's model of the cause of disease can also be used to help understand health in general.

Disease is literally a lack of ease. When the word is broken down, this is easy to see. Disease is usually associated with pain and dysfunction, two things that nobody wants. When the activity level of a tissue is normal, health and balance exist. As in the story of the Three Bears, the porridge desired is neither the one that is too hot nor the one that is too cold, but the one that is just right. A just-right tissue activity is associated with perfect health. Everyone knows about overactivity and underactivity in children. Either condition in a child is undesirable. Just the right amount of activity is what is normal and wanted. So it is with every cell in your body, every tissue, every organ, and indeed, every system. When a tissue is overfunctioning, it is called "acute," or "hyperactive." Conversely, when a tissue is underfunctioning, it is known as "chronic" or "hypoactive." (For graphic depictions of the four stages of tissue activity, see Figure 4.2.) Either way, a state of altered function exists. Altered function is a move to the right or left of center. Extended periods of abnormal function lead directly to a disease state, with, as a rule, symptoms to shortly follow. The breakdown of any organ—that is, reduced function—interferes with the function of every other organ in the body. This is the reason people say that one operation leads to another.

Overactivity is acute. Hyperactivity is usually synonymous with symptoms that make us feel ill at ease. Due to the acuteness, it is usually regarded as *dis*ease. Pain and discomfort are associated much more with hyperactivity than with hypoactivity, more with over-function than with under-function. Heat, redness, inflammation, fever, irritation, soreness, pus, drainage, discharge, and swelling all go along with hyperactivity of tissues. Unless underactive and chronic through heredity, tissues always become acute before they become chronic. This is the natural order of things. No one ever gave birth without first being pregnant.

An acute, inflamed condition is a necessary first step in the healing process. I'm wondering if you heard that! I'm going to

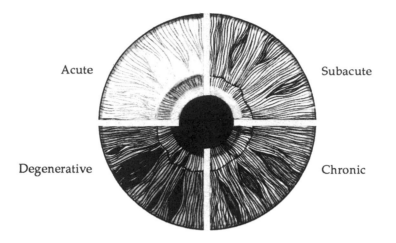

Figure 4.2. Above are the four stages of tissue imbalance—acute, sub-acute, chronic, and degenerative—viewed side by side. Below, the four stages, along with normal tissue, are shown as they appear in the iris fibers.

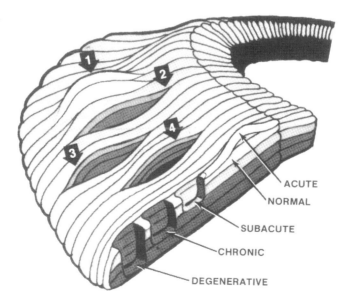

say it again. *Acute, inflammatory conditions are a necessary first step in the healing process.* Yet this is the precise time when temptation is the greatest to engage in acts of suppression. People want to *reduce* fever, swelling, pain, and inflammation, so they resort to all manner of drugs, nostrums, and potions in order to obtain a measure of relief. What many do not know is that all drugs do is suppress; they do nothing to help restore quality, healthy tissue. Drugs do not heal. Nature heals. Relief and suppressive measures do not correct the habits and lifestyles responsible for deteriorated health. Proper care of an acute condition in accord with nature's ways will arrest progression to the chronic stage of activity and assist in healing. Improper or suppressive care, and sometimes neglect, will encourage tissues to progress to a chronic condition. Although chronic conditions are more comfortable than are the acute stages of disease, they can be more destructive in the long run. And they are always more difficult to heal.

It is important to see that we *build* disease, going from one stage of inflammation to ever-more-chronic stages. If we do not take care of the initial stage of inflammation using corrective measures, we merely suppress our symptoms while we progress to a more chronic state. We eat, think, and live ourselves into deteriorating health. We can't have it both ways. We can't live on a diet of coffee and doughnuts and expect to build and maintain healthy tissue, any more than we can suppress ourselves into better health by the use of drugs.

Underactivity is chronic. Hypoactivity is associated more with lowered temperature in the affected area, stiffness, dull pain or no pain at all, loss of functional ability, lack of discharge or pus, and little, if any, swelling. Chronic conditions are more annoying than they are painful, but they are nonetheless serious. They develop from inherited weaknesses or from acute conditions that were not taken care of properly. The bulk of chronic conditions result from the latter.

If and when a condition is allowed to progress to the chronic and underactive stage, it generally becomes more difficult for a doctor to treat. Often, this is when the patient is told to learn to live with it. He has arrived at the point where the condition is managed rather than cured. Managing chronic conditions with suppressive drugs is very profitable for the pharmaceutical industry. The management of chronic disease brings in the greatest profits in medicine. But it is not restoration, it is not healing, and it is anything but a cure.

"Management of chronic disease" is a medical euphemism. It is not curing disease, but controlling it with the aid of suppressive drugs. This type of response to disease halts any progress toward healing. It serves only to make the patient more comfortable, while allowing him to progress to the degenerative stage, postponing the day of reckoning. Often, surgery is the last resort after years of neglect or suppression. Chronic conditions denied proper care will inevitably regress into ever-greater chronicity until they become degenerative. Degeneration is a severe degree of underactivity, at times even progressing to total tissue destruction. At this point, there is little, if any, functional ability left in the tissue. Failure of the organism to survive is the end result of degenerative conditions.

As we have seen, iridologists would rather express themselves in terms such as "overactivity" and "underactivity" of tissue than to name and classify disease. This is because the iris can tell the skilled iridologist whether tissues are in an overactive or underactive state. Iridology cannot tell if you have a stomach ulcer, but it can tell if the portion of your iris that reflexly represents your stomach is showing your stomach tissue to be overactive.

It is a cardinal tenet of iris analysis that its concern is mainly with determining the activity level of tissue and not with diagnosing or naming disease. Remember, normal functioning is never associated with any disease, pain, disability, or illness. Normal functioning is congruent with robust health. Healthy tissues are neither overactive nor underactive. They have just the right amount of activity. An iridologist need not resort to naming disease if he can determine if tissues are overactive or underactive, acute or chronic. This is how iridology understands the nature of disease, and this understanding is a prerequisite for iris analysis.

There you have it—a basic overview of iridology. As I have shown, iris analysis is a simple way of looking at the complex human organism. It tells a lot with a few basic tenets, tools, and signs. In Part Two, we will shuffle them all together and take a peek at iridology in action.

Part Two

A Peek at Iridology in Action

I believe there is more to be revealed in the iris than man will ever know.

—Dr. Bernard Jensen

5.

What Iridology Can and Cannot Show

Probably the question most frequently asked of an iridologist is, "What can you tell from looking at the iris?" It's certainly a fair question, even though no universal agreement exists among iridologists as to the meaning of *every* iris sign.

As you will see here in Part Two, where we take a look at iris analysis at work, not everything is directly presented in the iris as a particular iris sign. Frequently, an examiner must draw upon his understanding of anatomy, physiology, and clinical nutrition in order to correlate his interpretation of several iris signs. The experienced practitioner draws upon every aspect of his clinical experience in the course of making an iris analysis. Frequently, the iris is not the sole source of his information. The wise practitioner constantly attempts to correlate what he observes in the iris with other findings, as well as with any hunches or gut feelings he may have. To rely upon information gleaned from the iris alone is at least as risky as relying too heavily upon laboratory analysis, which is a habit many physicians have developed. Many types of tests and analysis procedures are extremely useful to the health practitioner, but they should be correlated with as much information from other sources as is practical.

In this chapter, I will present a list of what I believe iridology can show and a list of what I feel it can't show. Please notice when reading the list of things it can show that some of the statements may seem to overlap. I did this purposely to demonstrate that there is a close interrelationship between all the organs and systems in the body. There is often more than one way to look at a situation. For example, "Sources of infection" and "Where inflammation is located in the body" appear to be quite alike. What I am trying to bring out is that many times, a person may be harboring what is known as a "low-grade infection." A low-grade infection can be very difficult to locate and may be associated with subtle, yet annoying, symptoms. Laboratory blood tests, such as the erythrocyte sedimentation rate (ESR), an inflammation indicator, may not show elevation as they would with an outright inflammatory process. Although many infections are associated with an inflammatory process, the low-grade type may not result in enough inflammation to be clinically manifest. Iridology is a wonderful tool for finding the source of these low-grade, subclinical infections.

Some of the items on my lists are things about which iridologists are commonly questioned. A few are listed because other iridologists claim they can gain information about them, even though they have so far been unable to satisfactorily substantiate their claims. It is my sincere desire to list straightforwardly what I personally believe can and cannot be presently done. Please remember that it is quite possible, even probable, that continued research will lead to modification of these lists.

WHAT IRIDOLOGY CAN SHOW

My list of things that iridology can show is much longer than my list of things it can't show. And with continued research, as I just said, it should get longer.

So, without further ado, here are the things that I believe iridology can reveal.

- *The primary nutritional needs of the body.* Iridology can demonstrate the body's need for minerals, which are its chemical building blocks. Enzymes and vitamins promote chemical reactions in the body, but minerals are the raw materials from which body tissues are built. Dominant minerals are always in short supply in an inherently weak area.

- *The inherent strength or weakness of organs, glands, and tissues.* These are the areas most often in need of cleansing and directed nutritional support. Iridology is a science that evaluates relative inherent weaknesses and strengths.

- *Constitutional strength or weakness.* Iridology reveals the body's overall or average strength or weakness. People with a lesser number or degree of inherent weaknesses have a greater constitutional strength.

- *Which organs are in the greatest need of repair and rebuilding.* The organs in the greatest need are those that are the weakest, the most toxic, and in shortest supply of their dominant minerals.

- *The relative amount of toxic settlement in the organs, glands, and tissues.* The most toxic organs and tissues are the ones demonstrating the greatest degree of inherent weakness.

- *Where inflammation is located in the body.* Areas of inflammation are represented by an acute whiteness of the iris fibers.

- *The stage of tissue inflammation and activity.* This is shown by the degree of whiteness or darkness in the iris area representing the tissue.

- *Underactivity, or sluggishness, of the bowel.* This is represented in the iris by an inherently weak bowel area. The area may also exhibit ballooning, pockets, or both. Prolapsus (sagging) may also be evident. In addition, drug residues tend to settle in sluggish tissues as these tissues do not have the strength to throw them off. Plus, dominant minerals will probably be in short supply.

- *Spastic and ballooned conditions of the bowel.* A spastic condition is indicated when the autonomic nerve wreath moves very close to the pupil in the affected area. A ballooned condition is indicated when the nerve wreath moves farther away from the pupil in the affected area.

- *The need for acidophilus in the bowel.* Sluggishness, ballooning, and pockets in the bowel usually increase the transit time of bowel contents, allowing unfriendly bacteria to proliferate in the colon. Friendly acidophilus bacteria are needed to help restore the bacterial balance.

- *Prolapsus of the transverse colon.* Prolapsus is indicated by the upper horizontal section of the nerve wreath falling down, or sagging, toward the pupil.

- *A nervous condition or inflammation of the bowel.* This is indicated by the autonomic nerve wreath's structure and degree of whiteness. The wreath often appears to be raised in the acute area.
- *High-risk tissue areas in the body that may be progressing toward a disease.* Any area that is too white or too dark is a high-risk area. Both acute and chronic areas carry a degree of risk. Disease exists in both acute and chronic forms.
- *Pressure on the heart.* Bowel pockets in, or ballooning of, the transverse and/or descending colon, with attendant sluggishness and gas formation, are often responsible for pressure on the heart and reflex heart arhythmias.
- *The circulation level in various organs.* Underactive tissues have a decreased circulation and thus a lower temperature, whereas overactive, acute tissues have an increased circulation and elevated temperature.
- *Nerve force and nerve depletion.* Nerve force, which is nerve energy, and nerve depletion, which is lack of nerve energy, are judged largely according to the condition of the autonomic nerve wreath. Other factors also considered include the condition of the brain areas and of glands such as the adrenal, thyroid, and pituitary. (For a further discussion of nerve force, please see "Nerve Force," on page 77.)
- *Hyperactivity or hypoactivity of organs, glands, and tissues.* These can be acute, subacute, chronic, or degenerative, as evidenced by the degree of whiteness or darkness of the area's iris fibers.
- *The influence of one organ on another, or the contribution of an organ to a condition elsewhere in the body.* No organ stands alone. All organs are symbiotically related. The iris can sometimes reveal graphically how an acute or chronic area directly affects other tissues.
- *Lymphatic-system congestion.* The lymphatic rosary is a classic sign indicating widespread lymphatic congestion. However, certain areas of the body may display signs of congestive lymph without showing this more classical string-of-beads appearance.
- *Poor assimilation of nutrients.* This is seen in the assimilation

Nerve Force

To define "nerve force" is to attempt the impossible. Since man first found himself on the face of the Earth, he has pondered the essence of life. What is that special something that distinguishes the living from the dead, the animate from the inanimate? Can human life and energy be just the result of chemical oxidation? What is that special and unique force that is transferred by the nervous system? No one seems able as yet to fully answer these questions. But we continue to ponder them. It is the meat for philosophers and theologians.

Both Eastern and Western medicine have wrestled with the problem of nerve force, or nerve energy. In the East, the Chinese acupuncturists, with their philosophy of Taoism, call this special energy "Chi." They claim that it is Chi and its balance throughout the body that is activated or altered as the result of their therapy. Chi is tied to the great elemental forces of fire, Earth, air (wind), and water. Disturbances resulting in imbalances of this elemental energy in the body manifest as disease. The concepts are steeped in the mysticism of the Orient.

In the West, we like to think of ourselves as more scientific and less reliant on philosophers when we attempt to explain such an elusive concept as nerve force. In our attempt to elevate science to godhood, we often forget that our basic philosophical concepts originated in the Near East and are deep-rooted in our culture. The word "spirit" probably is the closest to the concept of Chi. "Spirit" is the English word that is the best translation for the Greek word "pneuma." If "pneuma" looks familiar, it's because it is the root of several English words, such as "pneumonia" and "pneumatic." You see, besides meaning "spirit," "pneuma" also translates into "air" or "wind." We are back to the elements again! We read in the Bible's creation stories that

> *God "breathed" into man the "breath of life." Once more, East meets West.*
>
> *I find it interesting that in modern times, the chiropractic profession uses the word "innate" to describe the unique nerve force that animates and enables life and healing. Chiropractic holds forth the concept that innate is responsible for healing and that proper spinal alignment facilitates the flow of innate by way of the nervous system. Call it what you will. I have chosen to use the term "nerve force."*

ring, at the interior pupilary margin.

- *Depletion of minerals in an organ, gland, or tissue.* Inherently weak tissues are always in need of their dominant minerals.
- *The relative ability of an organ, gland, or tissue to hold nutrients.* Inherently weak tissues cannot hold their nutrients as well as stronger tissues can.
- *The results of physical or mental fatigue or stress on the body.* Stress is indicated by nerve rings, or stress rings, in the iris. A pupil that is large and unable to contract quickly and adequately when exposed to light indicates chronic fatigue. Other signs, such as a dropped transverse colon and brain anemia, as well as a weak thyroid or adrenal glands, may also be associated with fatigue.
- *The need for rest to build up immunity.* Rest is the greatest healer there is. Immunity is lowered with fatigue. All sick people are fatigued and need rest.
- *Tissue areas contributing to suppressed or buried symptoms.* Chronic areas often contribute to more acute symptoms, as well as to lesser ones. The iris reveals acute, subacute, and chronic areas, which are sometimes difficult to detect or locate by standard examination procedures.
- *High or low sex drive.* Sex drive is often an indicator of other health problems. A fatigued person cannot have a normal sex drive. There is also a certain brain area that is connected with sex drive, with a weakness there sometimes causing continued low drive in a person of otherwise good health.

Of course, a heightened sex drive can also occur, although fewer people seem to complain about this.

- *A genetic pattern of inherent weaknesses and their influence on other organs, glands, and tissues.* Again, all organs and systems are related to one another. When one suffers, all are affected to some degree.

- *The effects of iatrogenic conditions.* Iatrogenic conditions are caused by the treatments of doctors. All drugs have side effects, some of which can be serious. The iris can reveal drug settlements.

- *The preclinical stages of diabetes, cardiovascular conditions, and many other diseases.* The iris can reveal subacute conditions and inherent weaknesses that often go unrecognized by other methods. Early attention is thus possible.

- *Miasms.* Miasms are a discoloration of the entire iris caused by putrid matter, toxins, and settlements accumulating in the tissues. (See Figure 3.9 in Chapter 3.) A miasmic eye is sometimes called a "dishwater eye" because its iris color resembles dirty dishwater. (For a further discussion of miasmic eyes, please see "The Miasmic Iris," on page 80.)

- *The recuperative ability and health level of the body.* These are shown by the constitution—the overall density—of the iris fibers.

- *The buildup of toxic material before the manifestation of a disease.* Toxic settlements are represented by an iris color that departs from the basic inherited color. All diseases are related to increased levels of toxic substances in the body.

- *Genetic weaknesses affecting the nerves, blood supply, and mineralization of bone.* Genetic weaknesses can affect any area, depending on location and severity.

- *The genetic influence on any symptoms present.* Problems, and thus symptoms, tend to occur in the areas of the greatest genetic, or inherited, weakness. These are the areas we should learn about and take care of before problems flare. Iridology is the only science that can reveal inherited weaknesses, indicating their degree and location.

- *Healing signs indicating an increase of strength in an organ, gland, or tissue.* A positive iris sign is the healing line, which indicates the repair and strengthening of tissues. It is a sign of new tissue replacing old.

The Miasmic Iris

"Miasm," or "miasma," is a word that stems from the Greek and means "pollution," "stain," or "defilement." In iridology, we speak of a "miasmic iris," or "miasmatic iris."

A miasmic iris appears dull, murky, and lackluster. (See Figure 3.9 in Chapter 3.) Its color can seem washed out, off-color. Because of this, the basic color of the iris may be difficult to define. I often call such an iris a "dishwater eye" because to me, its color looks like dirty dishwater: grayish, polluted, nondescript.

Before I continue, let me stress that although miasm is associated with inherited and acquired drug settlements, it should not be confused with the obvious color alteration also associated with drug settlements. This latter type of color alteration is most often confined to areas of relative inherent weakness, such as the bowel, represented inside the autonomic nerve wreath. Miasm, on the contrary, affects both irides and affects them in their entirety. It is in no way limited only to areas representing inherently weaker tissues. In addition, miasm is something more than just the simple drug settlements frequently found in inherent weaknesses. Miasm is more a blood pollution than a pollution of anything else. As a blood pollution, it influences all the tissues, disturbing brain activity, glandular function, and cellular metabolism.

Miasm, as I just mentioned, is associated with inherited and acquired drug settlements. The drugs include—yet are by no means confined to—pharmaceuticals and illicit drugs. Any substance entering the body by whatever means, and not of the nature of a natural and wholesome nutrient, can settle in the tissues and result in toxic pollution and irritation. When the body absorbs enough of these materials over an extended period, a miasmic iris can slowly manifest. In this regard, please note that normal metabolic activity produces its own toxic wastes and, should the major elimina-

tion systems be significantly underfunctioning, these "natural" noxious elements can also contribute to a miasmic condition.

Perhaps the most important consideration when dealing with miasm is that of suppression. The drugs and nostrums that our society freely uses to relieve the various symptoms of illness all have a suppressive effect. We must remember that drugs do not cure; they provide, at best, relief that is temporary. However, relief through drugs always has its price. Accompanying nearly all conditions is a mucous, or catarrhal, drainage. Catarrh contains putrid, toxic materials and is nature's avenue for eliminating these materials from the body. Suppression of catarrhal eliminations, although providing a measure of relief from discomfort, does not allow for the elimination of these toxic wastes, and their accumulation in the tissues thus continues.

As with catarrh, drugs, with their inherent side effects, contribute to a miasmic condition when not entirely eliminated from the body. Miasm can result in such a chronic irritation in the body that all the tissues are affected. Even the psychological state may be altered. I believe that miasm can be classified as a type of blood "dyscrasia." "Dyscrasia" is a medical term, again stemming from the Greek, meaning "bad temperament," a morbid condition, especially one involving imbalance.

People who have a miasm need to "clean up their act." They need to come clean both in their elimination and in their diet and lifestyle. Due to the suppressive and very chronic nature of miasm, the condition is difficult to remove completely. In my experience, people exhibiting miasmic irides need to cleanse their systems often, extensively, and repeatedly. This should include fasting, colon washing, diet modification, and use of certain homeopathic preparations and herbals, as well as permanent lifestyle change. With attention and resolve, a miasm can be improved. However, in very chronic and severe cases, I doubt if the manifestation can ever be removed entirely from the iris.

- *The potential for varicose veins in the legs.* Inherent weakness in the leg area of the iris indicates a potential for varicose veins to develop. Remember, inherent weakness does not necessarily indicate that there are, or will be, any clinical symptoms or overt manifestations. However, areas of relative weakness have more potential to develop problems than do inherently stronger areas.
- *Positive and negative nutritional needs of the body.* Settlements seen in the iris indicate that substances were taken into the body that could not be used as food. Similarly, inherent weaknesses reveal the need for additional nutrients.
- *A probable allergy to wheat.* When allergies are experienced, wheat is the first thing that comes to mind since it is such a common allergen. Acidity seen in the iris is often associated with too much wheat in the diet.
- *Sources of infection.* Locating the source of an infection is one of the most useful functions of iridology. Look for an acute or chronic area. Low-grade infections are usually chronic and difficult to locate without iridology.
- *Acidity of the body and catarrh development.* Over-acidity is indicated by an acute whiteness of the iris fibers in a blue iris and a light yellow color of the fibers in a brown iris. This is usually accompanied by increased mucous production and flow, which can lead to catarrh, an inflammation of the mucous membranes.
- *Suppression of catarrh.* The suppression of catarrhal discharges with drugs and nostrums can lead to a chronic or subacute condition.
- *The condition of tissues in any one part of the body, or in all the parts of the body at one time.* You can tell whether tissues are acute, normal, chronic, or degenerative in their activity.
- *The climate and altitude that are best for the patient.* An analysis of the patient's health problems, strengths and weaknesses, heart condition, etc., can help determine the best living conditions for him. Climate and altitude can have a distinct effect on certain health conditions.
- *The potential for senility.* Iris signs such as brain anemia, a cholesterol ring, and other indicators of compromised circulation can suggest current or potential senility.

- *The effects of a polluted environment.* Drug settlements can be associated with the environment as well as with the intake of medications. Intake can occur through the skin or from air, water, or food. Even the ears and eyes can take in pollution, in the form of sound and sight.
- *Adrenal exhaustion.* Adrenal exhaustion can indicate low blood pressure, lack of energy, slowed tissue repair, and deficiencies of vitamin C and adrenaline. Look at the adrenal area of the iris.
- *Resistance to disease.* The body's ability to resist disease correlates directly with the amount of toxic settlements in the body.
- *The relationship or unity of symptoms with conditions in the organs, glands, and tissues.* As stated before, everything in the body is related to everything else.
- *The difference between a healing crisis and a disease crisis.* Healing lines will be evident before a healing crisis occurs. Also, the bowel will function well during a healing crisis but not during a disease crisis.
- *The accuracy of Hering's Law of Cure.* All healing takes place from the head down, from the inside out, and in the reverse order from which the conditions were acquired. The truth of this law is witnessed every day by the iridologist.
- *Whether a particular program or therapy is working.* A program that is working will produce healing lines, a reduction in drug deposits, clarity of the iris, decreased acidity and catarrh, etc., while a wrong therapy will not. Do not let symptoms alone be your guide.
- *The quality of nerve force (nerve energy) in the body.* The indicators are the size of the pupil, the contraction and condition of the autonomic nerve wreath, and the condition of the brain areas.
- *The body's response to a treatment.* Iris analysis can reveal how well the body is healing itself and at what rate. Look for positive changes in the iris, including a lightening of color and the appearance of healing lines.
- *The whole, or overall, health level of the body.* Compare the tissue integrity of the different organs to one another. The average indicates the overall health level.

Iridology is a powerful tool. The presence of just one sign can reveal a multitude of conditions. Read back through this list to see just how many things each sign can indicate. And while you're taking your second look at the list, note how the absence of a sign can tell a glorious story, too.

WHAT IRIDOLOGY CANNOT SHOW

It may help you in our continuing examination of the science and art of iridology to learn that not unlike other diagnostic systems, there are limitations to what the iris can reveal. Some iridologists claim that they can tell certain things from examining the iris that I have not been able to substantiate. The following is a list of some of the things that I sincerely believe cannot be discerned. If anyone feels he can prove any of them otherwise, I stand ready to accept a demonstration to the contrary. I recognize that there is yet much more to understand about what is seen in the iris.

- *Blood pressure levels (normal or abnormal), blood sugar level, and other specific diagnostic findings and laboratory test results.* Iridology can reveal a lack or an excess, whether of a substance or a force, but not the specific amount.
- *Which specific medications or drugs an individual is using or has used in the past.* Years ago, when the drugs prescribed by physicians were simpler in their chemical structure, the iridologist could make a good guess as to which one had settled in the tissues by observing the iris color. For example, iron was rust colored, sulphur was yellow, and quinine was green. Modern drugs, however, are usually compound formulas. In addition, people today are more apt to have taken, or be taking, several drugs.
- *What surgical operations a person has had.* Scar-tissue formation can sometimes be noticed in the iris, thus suggesting surgical intervention, but this is usually not possible.
- *Specifically what foods a person does and does not eat.* Sometimes an iridologist can get a pretty fair idea of what general foods a person consumes, but this is not certain and it cannot be done for a specific food.
- *How much uric acid is in the body.* Although an iridologist can

tell if someone has too many noxious acids in his body, he cannot tell which specific acids are involved.

- *The time and cause of an injury to the body.* Iridology cannot show such specifics, although it can sometimes reveal that there was an injury.
- *Whether a snake bite is poisonous and if the snake venom has entered the bloodstream.* The effects of hundreds of snake bites over a lifetime may show up in the iris, but probably not of one or even just several.
- *The correlation between tissue-inflammation levels and specific diseases or symptoms of disease.* Iridology cannot diagnose disease.
- *Diseases by name.* Once again, iridology cannot name diseases.
- *Whether a subject is male or female.* The only clue you have is the mascara on the eyelashes!
- *Whether asbestos settlements or silicosis exist in the body.* Iridology cannot tell which specific elements have settled in the tissues.
- *If hair is falling out and why.* Falling hair is annoying, but it is not in itself a disease state of the body.
- *The number of organs with which a person was born.* Iridology cannot tell if a person was born with three kidneys, a double uterus, etc.
- *The presence of a yeast infection, such as Candida albicans.* Candida is a specific disease, which iridology cannot reveal. However, iridology can reveal conditions supporting its *possible* presence in the body.
- *Which tooth is causing problems.* Iridology cannot be so location-specific at this point in its development.
- *The presence of lead, cadmium, aluminum, or any other metallic elements in the tissues.* Iridology cannot tell which specific substances may have settled in the tissues.
- *If a woman is on birth control pills.* Again, iridology cannot reveal which specific medication or drug an individual is taking.
- *If a woman is pregnant.* Pregnancy is a normal physiological condition for women, not an abnormal tissue alteration.
- *Whether an operation is necessary.* This is a medical evaluation.
- *Whether a tumor is present and what size it is.* The iridologist

can often see the tissue alteration that is represented by a tumor, but he cannot tell whether it has manifested as a tumor or not.

- *Whether hemorrhage exists in the body or where it is located.* Hemorrhage, in itself, is not a tissue alteration.
- *The difference between drug side-effect symptoms and the symptoms of actual diseases.* Iridology cannot differentiate between symptoms.
- *Whether irregular menstrual periods are caused by the thyroid.* Although iridology cannot tell positively, it can point out an underactive thyroid gland and thus give a lead for further investigation.
- *The presence of multiple sclerosis, Parkinson's disease, or bubonic plague.* Iridology cannot name diseases.
- *Whether healing signs indicate a raising of the general health level.* Healing signs may be present in just one particular area and may not necessarily indicate a raising of the general health level.
- *The presence of syphilis, gonorrhea, or another sexually transmitted disease.* These are specific diseases, which iridology cannot name.
- *Orientation toward homosexuality.* Homosexuality is an alternate sexual orientation and does not involve abnormal tissue change.
- *The presence of AIDS.* AIDS (acquired immunodeficiency syndrome) is a condition resulting from a virus, and iridology cannot discern a virus.
- *The presence of gallstones or kidney stones.* A stone is not a tissue alteration.
- *Whether a cardiac artery is blocked.* Iridology can discern if a condition exists that would predispose a person to a blockage of this type, but it cannot find definitely that a blockage exists.

Not all iridologists will agree with my list of what iridology cannot show. I have, over the years, heard a number of claims made by different iridologists about what they could or could not tell. In nearly every case, however, I have not been able to personally substantiate these claims. This is not to say that these claims are not true. Any and all claims concerning iris analysis should always be scrutinized in the fairest possible way.

Iridology begs for honest, unbiased research. Perhaps the best way presently to scrutinize one iridologist's claim is to have other iridologists substantiate it in their clinical practice. I want to stress again the potential for more to be revealed in the iris than we can at present determine or perhaps even imagine. To discern these as-yet-unseen or unrecognized things, we need to develop new understandings about health, plus more highly sensitive and sophisticated equipment for iris analysis. I believe the computer and the new digital-based equipment will be great aides in this regard as we move into the twenty-first century.

Anything new always seems to be automatically opposed. How many people are trying to think of ways to prevent disease? How many are searching for how to create new tissue with perfect functioning ability? These are the work of the iridologist.

When it comes to the matter of health, we are all living on relief, rich and poor alike. Most doctors are in the business of providing relief. Drugs and nostrums are also geared to giving relief of symptoms. We need to switch our concern to correction and away from relief. Correction is easiest when a problem is found in its subacute stage. And correction should begin before any clinical symptoms arise and relief is needed. Most people seek relief out of desperation. They should learn how a disease is built and take care of things before they get into a desperate situation.

Disease often begins with a lack of mineralization in the tissues. A weakened tissue cannot resist disease as well as a healthy tissue can. Weakness is an invitation for a disease process to begin. But how are we to know about a mineral deficiency or a tissue weakness? We shouldn't wait until we have a waiting-room disease that requires extreme drugging or surgical intervention. This is why I say we need new thinking. Good health depends on every organ working at its normal level of activity. Who is thinking this way? If everyone is thinking alike, someone isn't thinking.

Much good has been said about iridology. Of course, there has been a lot of negative response also. Iridology invites response. It is open to research. However, very often, those people who are the most critical have done the least research. It's easy to be down on what you're not up on.

    Horatio: "But this is wondrous strange!"

    Hamlet: "And therefore as a stranger give it welcome. There are more things in heaven and earth, Horatio, than are dreamt of in your philosophy."

6.

Eyeing Elimination

We're coming into the homestretch now and it's time to move into gear. We've learned all about iridology's origins, tools, terms, signs, how's, why's, can's, and can'ts. Now it's time to mix them all together and see what we come up with.

In this and the next chapter, we will take a peek at iridology in action. We will begin with a discussion in this chapter of what the irides can tell us about our five main elimination channels, especially the all-important bowel. In Chapter 7, we will discuss what an iris analysis can reveal about our brain areas, spine, glands, and circulatory system.

Iridology can be very powerful. Let's see why now.

THE BOWEL IS KING

In the physical body, the bowel is king. This is due to its very powerful influence on our health. The bowel being king, let's take a quick tour of the royal chambers.

Nearly everyone knows that the bowel is the hollow tube extending from the stomach to the anus. Actually, the mouth, esophagus, and stomach itself, even though not a part of the bowel, can also be included if we refer to the entire length as the "digestive tract." Digestion begins in the mouth. Therefore, it would be more accurate to think of the digestive tract as beginning at the mouth and extending to the anus.

The digestive tract can be broken down into two basic parts: the small bowel and the large bowel. The small bowel begins at the exit from the stomach and is smaller in diameter than the large bowel. It is very convoluted, folding back upon itself many times in order to save space and squeeze into the abdominal cavity—its adult length is approximately twenty-one feet. It's called the "small bowel" not because of its length but due to its relatively small diameter of approximately one-and-a-half inches. By contrast, the large bowel, which begins at the ileocecal valve, is just a little more than five feet in length but is nearly two-and-a-half inches in diameter.

The large intestine is often called the "lower bowel," or "colon." We will consider the colon first. This structure begins with the section called the "cecum" and its three-inch-long, worm-like appendage known as the "appendix," labelled "append" on the iris chart. (See Figure 6.1.) Nearly everyone knows where the large bowel begins because of the proximity of the appendix, which is found in the lower right abdominal region. Next comes the ascending colon ("ascend. colon" on the chart), so named because it ascends toward the liver on the right side of the abdomen. The colon then makes a left turn and, following this turn, or flexure, it becomes known as the "transverse colon." The transverse colon ("trans. c." on the chart), true to its name, continues transversely, or horizontally, left across the upper abdomen to just below the spleen, where it again makes a turn, this time downward. Because this turn occurs near the spleen, it is known as the "splenic flexure."

Following the splenic flexure, the colon is called the "descending colon" ("descend. colon" on the chart) because it indeed descends on the left side of the abdomen and proceeds toward the groin. There it makes yet another turn, called the "sigmoid flexure," after which this portion of the lower bowel is known as the "sigmoid colon." The large bowel then proceeds a short distance to the final turn in its journey, the rectal flexure. As expected, following this turn is the final section of the bowel, the rectum, which terminates with the anus. The anus has a powerful circular, or sphincter, muscle that when relaxed, allows evacuation of the bowel.

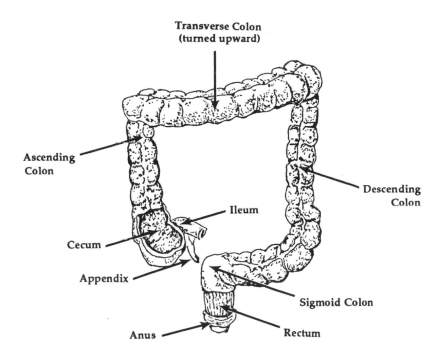

Figure 6.1. In iridology, the bowel is king. Above is a healthy large intestine, also known as the "lower bowel" or "colon."

The bowel has another important structure that bears mentioning. It is a special muscle with a kind of flap that acts like a butterfly check-valve, allowing intestinal contents to pass in one direction but not in the reverse. It's located where the small and large bowels meet, just before the appendix. It is the ileocecal valve. The function of this gate is to prevent reflux of intestinal contents from the large bowel back into the small intestine. In certain types of digestive disorders, it fails to function properly. Chronic constipation associated with improper diet and bowel habits, as well as with surgical removal of the appendix, often causes this valve to function incorrectly.

Every section of the intestinal tract has a particular function that contributes to the smooth operation of the organ as a whole. All in all, the total length of this biological plumbing approaches thirty feet.

Digestive-tract function is anything but simple. At this time, we don't need to concern ourselves with it. Anyone interested in learning the details can consult a comprehensive physiology text. I would like to point out, however, that the small bowel's major purpose is to prepare ingested foodstuffs for absorption. It facilitates the absorption of nutrients into the circulation, whereby sustenance is supplied to every cell in the body. The large bowel's main functions are to form and store the waste materials associated with the digestive process and, in due time, to expel them from the body. In so doing, it also helps to maintain the body's proper water balance. These are very elementary descriptions of the functions, but they will suffice for our purposes.

In iridology, we say that the bowel is king because it reigns over the entire body, its biological kingdom. It also occupies a large area on the iris chart. Take a look at the chart (Figure 2.1 on page 22–23) for a moment. Notice that the area depicting the bowel is second in size only to the combined brain areas. Notice also that the bowel is depicted in a ring formation around the pupil and that radially, from its scalloped periphery (the autonomic nerve wreath), extend nearly all the other organs of the body, not unlike the spokes of a wheel. This masterfully illustrates an anatomical phenomenon, as we shall soon see. This hub-like position around the pupil that is occupied by the bowel on the iris chart is why the bowel reigns over the entire body.

The story of the bowel's kingship is rooted in the history of our anatomical development. To learn how the king gained his kingdom, we should briefly examine our embryological development.

During the first month following conception, there are some fantastic developments in the new embryo. If these developments weren't real, they would be dynamite fiction. Biology students everywhere can name one of the first. It is the so-called "primitive gut tube." The primitive gut tube is the earliest visualized structure and, in time, will develop into the intestinal tract.

Sometime around the fourth week, as part of the normal developmental process, the newly forming digestive tract begins to sprout buds from its wall. These buds push out like branches from a tree trunk. As they grow longer and larger, they actually take the form of organs, such as the liver, pancreas ("pan." on the iris chart), lungs ("lung" on the chart), and bladder. Even the organs of the neck, such as the thyroid gland, larynx, and pharynx, are outgrowths of the digestive tract. Is it possible that organs can sprout from the intestines? Truth is stranger than fiction, they say.

Because of this outgrowth, these organs are actually encased in tissue that was once part of the intestinal wall. As development continues, the names change. The membrane covering the organs in their final development becomes known as the "parietal peritoneum" and covers the organs like a glove. Remember, developmentally, this is tissue from the bowel wall. And the organs, in their sprouting from the gut tube, drag along the nerves that are buried within the gut-tube walls. In this way, they maintain some of their original communication links with the digestive tract. Could this developmental history explain why irritations in the bowel reflexly influence organs opposite these areas, as depicted on the iris chart?

As I think of this marvelous developmental process, I am reminded of the motion picture *Gigi*. Here is the story of a young girl's development into a woman. As time passes, an aging Maurice Chevalier sees the little-girl-turned-young-woman and croons, "Gigi, am I a fool without a mind, or have I simply been too blind to realize it's you?" Although the little girl has developed into a young woman and is a new Gigi in many ways, she is still the same "little girl I used to know." In like manner, the organs change as they mature, but they keep—and we are reminded of—their developmental heritage. Much later in life, as different as they may then appear in the fullness of time, they still haven't entirely severed their developmental connections with what has become the adult intestinal tract. They're the "same Gigi" and still a part of the king's domain.

Look at the iris chart again. Find the ear and neck areas at about the 1:30 position in the left iris and at about 10:30 in the right iris. Can you find the descending colon area in the left iris and the ascending in the right iris, just opposite the ear and neck areas? Do you suppose that an irritation of the colon wall in either of these areas can affect the neck or ear? Can you see how an irritation of an intestinal area can affect the organ or area just opposite it on the chart? If you see this, you have learned one of the greatest concepts in iridology.

Let's examine another common bowel relationship. Can you see how an irritation midway down the descending colon can affect the heart via the nervous system? Do you think it could also affect the bronchial tubes ("bronchials") and lungs ("lung")? If you see these relationships on the iris chart, you are well on your way to understanding why iridologists say that the bowel is king. And you're also getting the idea of what makes iris analysis the wonderful art that it is.

The bowel is king because whenever the integrity of its tissues is compromised, it can—and usually does—have an effect on the organ areas opposite, as seen on the iris chart. I call this relationship the "neuro-arc syndrome." By the same token, when the intestinal tract is healthy and functioning well, the body as a whole tends to be well. When the intestinal tract is compromised in its tissue integrity, it can affect almost any area of the body. The iris chart confirms this. It is why, in iridology, we bow to the bowel as we would before a king.

BECOMING BOWEL-MINDED

Now it is time to recall Hering's Law. Do you remember it? It is: *All cure starts from within out, from the head down, and in the reverse order as the symptoms appeared.* The first step in the healing process is to take care of our insight, our attitude. This is represented by the pupil. It's the way we see things. The second step in the order, proceeding outward on the chart, is to take care of our intestinal tract. This includes improving our diet and our assimilation of nutrients. Inherent in this is taking care of our nervous system, represented by the bordering nerve wreath. If we take care of these three things—our brain (thoughts), bowel (the king), and nervous system—we have the master keys to health, healing, and long life. There is nothing in iridology that is more important than these three. Hering's Law teaches us through iridology that as we take care of our mind, bowel, and nervous system—especially the bowel—we help take care of everything else.

I can't begin to tell you about the marvelous success I have had with patients by just taking care of the bowel. Of course, let's not forget that this includes the diet also. The bowel is usually abused by our faulty dietary habits. If we desire health, we must straighten ourselves out in the eating department as part of our regular bowel care. I would like to share with you a story—my story—of how I personally learned about the kingship of the bowel.

A few years ago, I began to notice an increasing stiffness and aching in my left hip joint. I had no history of arthritis symptoms and was troubled over this new and persistent discomfort. I decided to visit a colleague to see if he could help me. He is a chiropractor, well-known in his profession and very capable. He took x-rays and did a quite thorough and wonderful diagnostic workup on me. When nothing outstanding showed up, he was puzzled. The good doctor gave me some therapy, which included specific manipulation for the hip to ensure proper range of motion and joint function. But in spite of what was masterful therapy, I still had the discomfort.

I knew from examining my irides that I had a bowel pocket, or diverticula, sign in my left iris, just opposite the left hip area. (See Figure 6.2.) This was in the region of the sigmoid colon, that portion of the colon just before the rectal area. Even though I knew it was there, I hadn't thought about it for quite some time. Often, a little discomfort can stimulate recollection. I therefore made arrangements to have a lower gastrointestinal (GI) series, which is also known as a "barium enema." Filling the colon with barium, a dense mineral, lets the colon's outline be visualized on x-ray. What do you think I saw when I looked at those films? I saw a bowel pocket, or diverticula, in the colon in the exact spot my iris indicated.

I showed these films to my colleague and suggested that I take care of my bowel. I told him that because of my work in iridology, I believed my bowel was causing my hip trouble. The good doctor, in return, tendered the thought that I was becoming "bowel-minded." He pointed out that over the years he had known me, he saw me become more and more concerned with the bowel. Well, I guess maybe I was bowel-minded. I had been lead—or perhaps I should say "driven"—to that position by seeing so many patients respond favorably to bowel care. Therefore, I decided to take extra good care of my bowel and my diet.

Wouldn't you know? My hip symptoms completely disappeared, returning only when I fail to give proper attention to my bowel. What I was experiencing in my own body was once again confirming what I had observed in my iridology work.

Another story I can relay to you is from my associate, Dr. Donald Bodeen. It concerns a young woman who visited Dr. Bodeen because he had helped her grandmother. Her problem was not one that would normally lead a person to a chiropractor. Her complaint was that she suffered episodes of abnormal heartbeat. When this happened, she feared for her life. She had been to several medical doctors and had even been hospitalized for tests. Although the arhythmias had been confirmed, the cause could never be determined. She didn't know what to do.

When Dr. Bodeen looked into her irides, he immediately noticed that she had a large, distended, and very chronic descending colon. It was quite dark, revealing a severe degree of chronicity. Dark, dirty bowel pockets and colon distentions usually indicate a lazy colon. In the lazy colon, bowel transit time is increased, fecal matter accumulates, and noxious colon bacteria produce fermentation and gas. Bowel transit time is the time it takes for ingested food to pass through the intestinal tract and out of the body. It can be checked by eating whole-kernel corn and noting how long it takes for the kernels to appear in the stool. Transit time should not exceed eighteen hours. Bowel gas always comes with chronic, dirty bowel pockets and distentions. In turn, the gas causes pressure to build. This pressure contributes to further distention. This is a vicious circle of degeneration.

Fermentation, pressure, and the associated toxic by-products irritate nerves in the colon wall and reflexly influence the organs located opposite them on the iris chart. As mentioned, I call this reflex influence the "neuro-arc syndrome."

Please recall that the heart area is located in the left iris, on the autonomic nerve wreath, just opposite the descending colon. If you look at the chart, you can see how gas pressures and chronic, or degenerative, areas in the descending colon can reflexly contribute to heart disturbances. Workers in any hospital emergency room will confirm that many people are rushed in thinking they are suffering a heart attack, only to find, after careful examination, that their symptoms are being caused by gas pressures. They are sent home, relieved, but still ignorant about diet and other preventative measures that can keep the condition from returning. Unfortunately, they are not taught about the need for, or ways to, take care of their bowel. If doctors would spend more time teaching their patients about diet and proper bowel care, they could spend less time trying to patch up the inevitable consequences of long-term neglect.

Because of what Dr. Bodeen observed in the iris of his young "heart" patient, he immediately suggested that she take care of her digestive system, including starting a diet and a program of bowel cleansing. He acquainted her with my *Ultimate Tissue Cleansing Program.* (For a description of the program, please see "The Ultimate Tissue Cleansing Program," on page 98.) After following this program and modifying her diet, the young woman happily confirmed that she had never felt better. Her heart symptoms had disappeared immediately and, to date, have not returned. It's cases like this that drive a person to become bowel-minded.

I would like to say that my associate, Dr. Bodeen, his wife, Joyce, and others who have joined me in this bowel work have witnessed remarkable results with patients who have done nothing more than take care of their bowel. My book describing the Ultimate Tissue Cleansing Program, *Tissue Cleansing Through Bowel Management*, details many of our cases and the wonderful results we have seen. Again, this is all because of the close and special relationship that the digestive tract has with the rest of the body.

Colon cancer is another bowel problem and it is on the rise. It is second only to malignancies of the breast and lung, and it likely will surpass lung cancer if the trend continues. Is it any wonder that 80 percent of bowel cancers are found in just three areas of the bowel, namely the cecum, the sigmoid, and the rectum? Iridologists are not surprised since these are the areas where the greatest number, the largest, and the dirtiest bowel pockets are found. These areas are the most toxic parts of the digestive tract when they show dirty pockets. Cancer is a chronic degenerative disease. The American Cancer Society tells us that it usually takes many years to develop a cancerous

The Ultimate Tissue Cleansing Program

The Ultimate Tissue Cleansing (UTC) Program is exactly what its name suggests. The bowel is the body's single most important system of elimination. We eliminate about two pounds of toxic wastes daily via the bowel. Because the bowel is king and all the other organs and systems can only be as clean as the bowel, an ultimate tissue cleansing is effected only by cleansing the bowel. I have found through my work in iridology and experiences at the ranch that the bowel is always in need of attention. When it gets proper attention, the whole body improves.

To cleanse the bowel, there are several things that we must do. We must improve our diet. We cannot cleanse our bowel while eating a diet that is improper. If our diet consisted of only a wide variety of pure, organically grown, wholesome, unadulterated foods, eaten raw or properly prepared, we would have little need for programs such as the Ultimate Tissue Cleansing Program. But tell me, who can live this way in our world today? Very few indeed! The truth is that we now live in a world with increasingly polluted air, water, and soil. Even space, the last pristine frontier, is becoming polluted.

We can expect maximum results from a cleansing or detoxification program only if we fast as an integral part of the program. From day one of the six-day UTC intensive, our ingestion is limited to the allocated supplements and cleansing drinks, plus water and an occasional cup of herbal tea or vegetable broth. This not only allows the carefully selected supplements to do their cleansing work, but also gives our digestive tract a physiological rest. Healing is accelerated by regular periods of rest. If we never fast, our

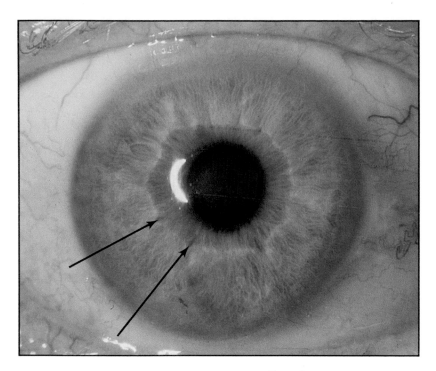

Bowel pocket

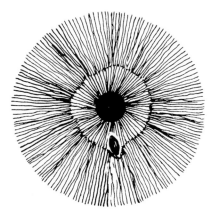

Figure 6.2. A bowel pocket, or diverticula, is a little pocket, or indentation, in the side of an intestine where waste material can accumulate. The waste material can cause many annoying problems.

Plate 10   *Visions of Health*

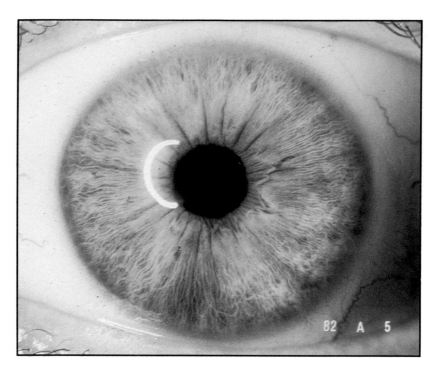

Radii solaris

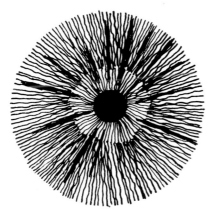

Figure 6.3. Radii solaris look like their name, rays of the sun. They seem to act as a trough that allows toxins to seep from one area to another. They are most common in the area between 11:00 and 1:00.

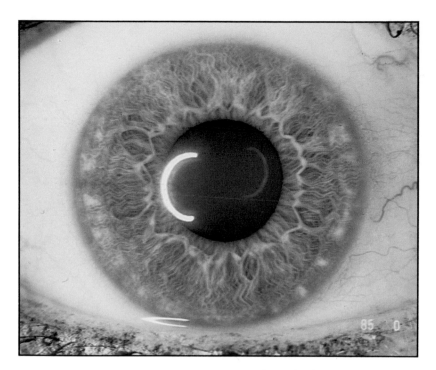

Lymphatic rosary

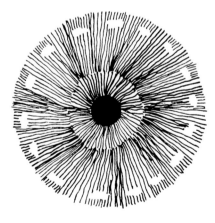

Figure 6.4. A lymphatic rosary is a string of cottony-appearing puffs that indicates heavy lymphatic-system congestion. The lymphatic system is a major elimination system in the body.

Plate 12   *Visions of Health*

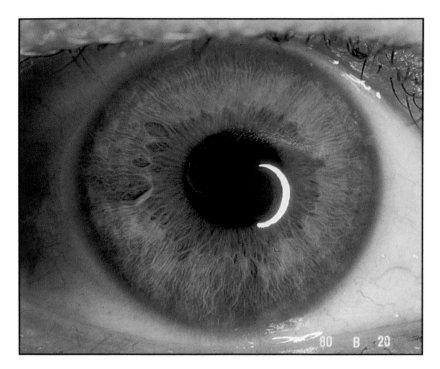

Scurf rim

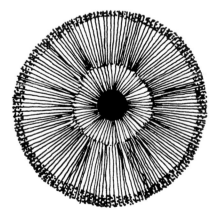

Figure 6.5. A dark rim around the iris, in zone 7 and possibly extending to zones 6 and 5, is a scurf rim. It indicates problems with the elimination of toxins through the skin.

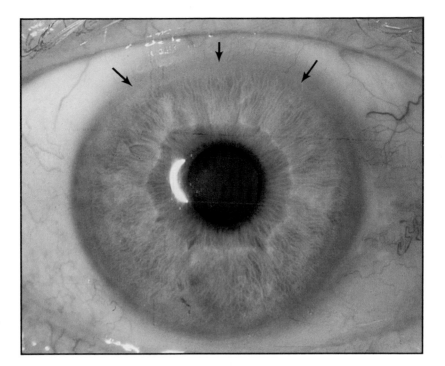

Arcus senilis

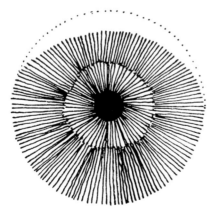

Figure 6.6. A major circulatory indicator is the arcus senilis, or arc of old age. It is a crescent-shaped sign in the brain areas, usually in zone 7, and indicates compromised circulation to the brain.

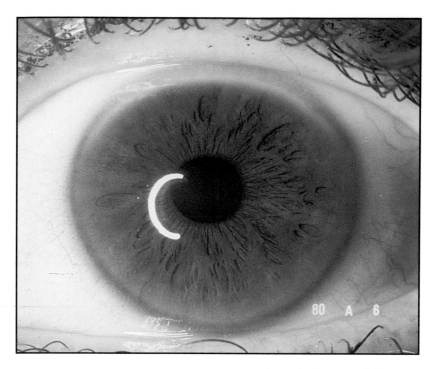

Anemia in extremities

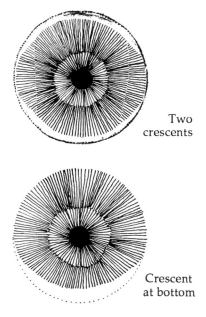

Two
crescents

Crescent
at bottom

Figure 6.7. The anemia in
extremities sign represents
compromised circulation to
the brain and other extremities. It can appear as a crescent in the upper portion of
the iris, the lower portion, or
both simultaneously. When
at the top, it is known as the
"arcus senilis" (see Figure
6.6).

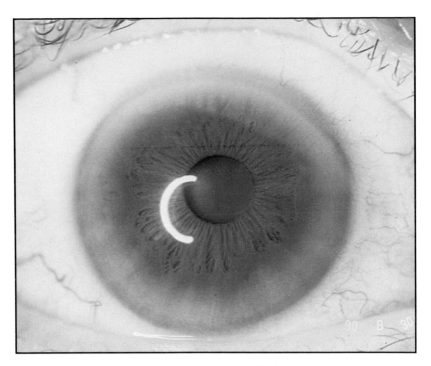

Sodium ring

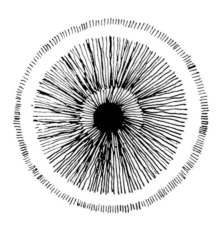

Figure 6.8. A sodium ring, or cholesterol ring, indicates heavy sodium intake and high blood-cholesterol levels. It is a milky-white ring in zones 6 and 7.

Plate 16 *Visions of Health*

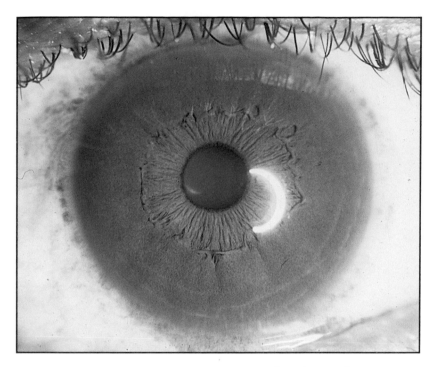

Circulatory ring

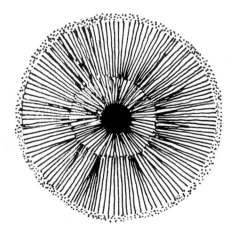

Figure 6.9. The circulatory ring appears as a bluish-purple ring on the peripheral side of zone 7 when venous return of the blood is hampered. It indicates that conditions are right for varicose veins to develop.

digestive system becomes the only part of our body that never rests. Think about it! Even our heart rests between beats.

Along with fasting, the UTC regimen employs colon washing. We refer to this cleansing as a "colema." The word "colema" is a combination of "colonic" and "enema." The colema is a special kind of colon cleansing. It is much more effective and a lot easier than an enema, without the high cost, complicated equipment, and other disadvantages commonly associated with colonics. The equipment consists of a plastic-coated colema board, a five-gallon bucket, surgical rubber tubing, and a rectal tip. It is relatively inexpensive to purchase, easy to use, and easy to clean. Personal ownership and use eliminate any possibility of cross-contamination. And in addition to being easy to use and sanitary, it is actually pleasant to use.

On the program, the colon is cleansed morning and evening, each session using five or more gallons of water with a liquid clay, chlorophyll, or coffee additive. During the week-long program, participants usually rest, read, watch educational video tapes, listen to audio tapes, and go for walks. At the conclusion of the program, the fast is broken with a simple, wholesome breakfast, followed by a resumption of what is hopefully an improved diet.

Colon washings (colemas) can also be instituted any time after the program is completed. In addition, the program as a whole should be repeated after eight weeks of following an improved diet and healthier lifestyle. The number of repetitions necessary to affect maximal cleansing varies with age, general health, the chronicity of problems, and the effort put into a total program of right living.

For more information about the Ultimate Tissue Cleansing Program and for details on how to obtain colema apparatus and supplies, please see "For More Information," on page 157.

condition. It is a well-known fact that tissues may be in a precancerous state for quite some time before progressing to a full-blown malignancy.

Not many years ago, cancer authorities and organizations were discounting the role of diet in cancer prevention and treatment. They said that diet had nothing to do with the development of cancer and was useless in its treatment. I can hardly believe the change that has recently come about in these same people and organizations. Increasingly, they are telling us that diet indeed plays a major role in reducing the chance of developing certain cancers, not the least of which is cancer of the bowel. We should take heed. Be assured, much more information will come from the authorities in the days ahead as the research of allopathic medicine continues in its enlightenment.

In your iris examination of the bowel areas, look for underactive, dark spots just inside, and bordering, the nerve wreath. They represent diverticulae, or bowel pockets, and when they are dark, they are underactive, dirty, and an irritant to the nerves in the bowel wall. They may—and likely will—irritate the area appearing opposite them on the iris chart. You will find the majority of these dirty pockets in the left iris, in the descending colon and sigmoid colon. But you will also find them in the right iris, usually in the area of the ascending colon. Again, remember the neuro-arc syndrome.

Generally, the descending and sigmoid colons are always a little darker than the rest of the intestinal areas. As mentioned, this is because the greatest number of darkened bowel pockets are usually found here. These areas are where diverticulae form. It is common to find dark, pocketed areas near the flexures, or bends, in the intestine, especially in the sigmoid colon. In this regard, let me mention that many children who have chronic ear problems or mastoid conditions also have trouble in the flexure opposite these areas on the chart.

Don't forget to look for healing lines in these dark bowel pockets. If healing lines are evident, ask your subject if he had any problems in the area that is now showing improvement.

Without the benefit of an iris analysis, many patients are mistakenly treated for their symptoms rather than for the physical cause of their problems. When you finally see the intimate cause-and-effect relationship between the bowel and the remainder of the body, you, too, will be on the road to becoming bowel-minded. Bowel-mindedness is a mark of the knowledgeable iridologist. Always be on the lookout for this relationship in every iris you examine. I consider the intimate relationship of the bowel to the areas opposite it on the iris chart to be one of my greatest discoveries in iridology.

RAYS OF THE SUN

There is another iris sign that is often functionally linked with the bowel. Iridologists refer to this sign as "radii solaris," which means "rays of the sun." Radii solaris are usually spoken of in the plural since in most irides where they are manifest, they are nearly always in multiples.

Rays of the sun are so named because of their appearance. If you imagine the pupil of the eye as being a sun, then these signs closely resemble the rays extending outward, as in drawings of a sun made by children. (See Figure 6.3.) Frequently, the rays extend out from the bowel area. In some irides, they begin a little farther out and extend perhaps half or three-quarters of the way to the periphery. When displayed, they are always more concentrated in the region between 11:00 and 1:00 in both eyes.

Radii solaris appear darker than their surrounding tissues. In fact, they are chronic inherent weaknesses in the tissues in which they are located. They are more significant when they begin at or inside the nerve wreath than when they are further removed from the wreath. Sometimes, they begin near the pupilary margin. Some iridologists refer to the ones that begin inside the wreath as "radii solaris major" and to the ones that begin farther out as "radii solaris minor." Those beginning within the bowel area—that is, inside the wreath—seem to facilitate the seepage of toxins from the bowel into the blood. As always, these toxins tend to settle in the weakest areas, in this case the areas into which the radii solaris extend. The radii solaris almost seem to act as a trough, or conduit, for toxins.

A person having a number of heavy, dark radii solaris extending from the bowel area into the brain areas is prone to such symptoms as toxic headaches, dulled thinking, sinusitis, slowness of mental faculties, mental stupor, and lack of concentration and retention. These are especially noticeable when the person has a chronic toxic bowel or is constipated. The person must strive to stay on a good diet and to pay special attention to his bowel function to minimize or avoid these toxic-related conditions. This holds particularly true if the bowel—specifically the transverse colon—is pocketed and itself suffers a compromised tissue integrity.

Part of becoming bowel-minded is to look for these radii solaris and to see them as the toxic conduits that they are. With proper care, radii solaris can, like all tissues, be upgraded in integrity. As this happens, they will become lighter. However, they will never completely disappear. They are like a crease, or fold, in a piece of paper. Even if you fold the paper back on itself in an attempt to remove the crease, the crease line will still remain. You may get the paper quite flat again, but the fold will always be visible. Likewise with radii solaris. Although an inherent weakness can be cleansed of toxic settlement and somewhat strengthened, it can never be as strong as genetically, or inherently, stronger tissues.

Look for radii solaris in every iris. Try to distinguish the major ones from the minor ones. Once again, the major type extend through the wreath into the bowel area, sometimes nearly to the pupilary margin, while the minor type are confined to the areas outside the wreath. Both types can appear in the same iris. Remember, all else being equal, the less there are, the better the constitution. And the lighter they are, the less toxic they will be and the less they will influence the organs into which they extend.

THE FIVE MAIN ELIMINATION CHANNELS

Cleanliness is next to godliness, they say. I find there is truth in this statement, especially regarding the mind and body. The average person believes that keeping clean consists of taking a shower and using the right deodorant. This is nice for the exterior of the body, but true cleanliness, like beauty, is more than skin deep.

Again harking back to Hering's Law, we see that we must

work *from within out* and *from the head down.* Cleanliness therefore begins with clean thoughts. A dirty person has dirty
thoughts. Filth can be as much of the mind as of the body. We
must be clean within our deepest self. Otherwise, we will learn
firsthand how one type of filth breeds another. Proceeding
outward from here on the iris chart, we come to the absorption
ring, the stomach, the bowel, and so on. Notice that according
to the chart, taking care of the skin is the last thing to do, but
certainly not the least. Do you remember this journey? We have
taken it before. It is travelling from the inside outward, according to Hering's Law.

Our cleanliness is in part determined by what we digest.
Our thinking may be food for thought, but our culinary habits
determine the food on our table. What I am suggesting here is
as simple as clean living with regard to what we eat. Making a
habit of eating the wrong kinds of food can create an unclean
environment internally. Today, there is much ado about clean-
ing up the environment, which has been polluted by man's
carelessness, neglect, and greed. We have brought ecological
disaster upon planet Earth. But it should be affirmed that we
have a personal ecology too, an internal environment to care for
and keep pollution-free.

There are five main avenues through which the body rids
itself of toxic waste products and keeps its internal ecology in
balance. We just spent the first half of this chapter discussing
the king of all the elimination channels, the colon. Before we
leave that old friend, let me just throw in a few parting
thoughts.

Nearly everyone should find it obvious that the colon is the
main sewer system of the body. The lower bowel's chief function
is to store and excrete solid wastes. Yet, it's amazing how many
people give little or no thought to this daily function. When we
consider thought, we again come to the importance of the mind
and brain. The bowel is often considered to be a dirty subject
and is thus excluded from the mind as well as from conversation. I have a few patients who can't remember if they had
a bowel movement yesterday—or even today—but they can
name every item they purchased on a shopping trip last week.
They would do better to pay greater attention to what they
should be getting rid of instead of focusing on what they have

acquired. They need to become bowel-minded in order to achieve better health.

Chronic constipation is a national health problem. Laxatives are second in over-the-counter drug sales, trailing only pain relievers such as aspirin and acetaminophen. And, in the United States, we swallow about 33 billion aspirin each year. A person cannot be constipated and maintain a clean inner environment. In fact, digestive diseases of all kinds are associated with constipation. Chronic constipation is nearly always at the root of digestive troubles. Every day, 200,000 Americans stay home from work because of a digestive-tract illness. One person in every ten in the United States has a chronic digestive disease. Half the population suffers occasional digestive distress. Digestive complaints are the leading cause of hospitalization and surgery. About 200,000 people in the United States die each year from diseases of the digestive system. There are over 100 diseases of the digestive system, most linked in some way with a history of chronic constipation or lack of proper bowel care, including diet. Lack of proper bowel care, resulting in poor bowel function, is the single greatest cause of disease and health troubles I know. *According to my experience, everyone has a chronic bowel problem to some degree, even if strongly denied.* My associate, Dr. Bodeen, would agree with me that 100 percent of the patients coming into nearly any doctor's office have bowel problems contributing in some manner to their ill health.

Look to the bowel first when you examine an iris. It was none other than Hippocrates, the father of medicine, who admonished his students to look to the bowel first. As a matter of interest, the very word "physician" comes from the word "physic." This is because early physicians looked to the bowel first and often gave a physic to move the bowel as the first treatment. What do today's physicians do? They neglect the bowel! Look back at Chapter 3 for some of the things you should try to observe in the intestinal area. The wise iridologist always looks to the bowel first. He knows that the bowel is king.

Next in the line of major elimination systems moving from the inside out are the bronchi and bronchial tubes. The bronchi are the two large, main air tubes going into the lungs. They divide into many small branches, the bronchials. The bronchials look like the branches of a tree as they extend deep into the lungs. In fact, this system resembles a tree so much that it is often called the "bronchial tree." It is in the smaller branches of this tree that much of the trouble starts, caused by old, chronic mucous accumulations. This is where bronchial pneumonia and bronchitis occur. Although these can be acute conditions, they are brought on by chronic degeneration that is associated with faulty diet and poor living habits. Inherent weakness in the bronchus, bronchials, and lung areas can be seen by the iridologist and is nearly always associated with these chronic problems. And, as we have noted time and again, mucous and toxic wastes always settle first, and in the greatest amounts, in tissues with lowered integrity.

Look for an inherent weakness in the bronchus, bronchials, and lung areas as you examine the iris. Remember, a darkened area indicates the development of a chronic condition, whereas white fibers within a darkened area indicate an acute condition. As always, look out for healing lines. You will see far more chronic conditions than acute conditions in the iris. As with the bowel, you will find that nearly every iris displays a chronic condition in these respiratory areas. It's estimated that over 187 million people in the United States have a disease in some stage of progress. That's almost eight out of ten people. That's why you'll definitely find these iris signs if you look for them.

The next organ of elimination to be considered is the kidney. Just as we have two lungs and two bronchi, we are endowed with two kidneys. This is because these organs are so very important to life. The kidneys' chief function is to purge the blood of toxic waste products and then eliminate the toxins through the urine. The iridologist considers the kidneys to be one of the five main elimination systems.

Not unlike the bowel, lungs, and bronchials, the kidneys are a common site of inherent weakness and lowered tissue integrity. Fortunately, as with our lungs, we do not use our kidneys to capacity. People can, and do, live on one kidney without undue health complications. A few people are born with only one functioning kidney. The tremendous reserve filtration of two kidneys allows a certain degree of inherent weakness and dysfunction to exist in the kidneys without a person manifesting symptoms of toxic blood.

As I already mentioned, it is not unusual to visualize a

rather marked compromise of kidney integrity in the irides of most people. Standing alone, this lowered integrity may not be a cause for immediate concern. However, if the condition is in addition to compromised function and lowered integrity of other major elimination systems, things can add up. When one elimination system is experiencing a significant degree of dysfunction, the other elimination systems must compensate; they each must work harder to carry their share of the added load. You can readily see the problem that develops when several major elimination systems fail to function optimally. This is when symptoms begin. Most people have subclinical, or even outright, manifestations of an elimination deficit associated with lowered tissue integrity in more than one major elimination system. I hope you can see why the iridologist gives his greatest attention to the organs and systems of elimination.

Look in the iris for evidence of inherent kidney weakness. Weaknesses may be manifest in one or both kidneys. Are the areas of inherent weakness very dark and chronic? Do radii solaris extend into the kidney area? Do nerve rings traverse the kidney? Are heavy drug settlements present? As always, don't forget to look for healing lines. Inherent weakness in the kidneys is common. You should not have any trouble finding some good examples.

The lymphatic system, designated "lymphatic and circulatory systems" on the chart, is another main elimination system and a major component of a larger system that has recently come into the public eye. With the advent of AIDS, the immune system has been thrust into the spotlight. It is the body's defense department. As a major component of the immune complex, the lymph system, as it is called, plays a leading role in this defense activity. Like blood, lymph fluid is both a nutrient provider and a waste collector. It circulates in very small, thin-walled conduits that reach into the most inaccessible depths of the organism. This clear, very thin liquid goes where blood cannot go. For instance, it can go into the lens of the eye, which it supplies with nutrients and cleans of cellular waste products. Because it is clear, we can look right through it. Lymph fluid is actually more like a gas than a liquid because it reaches places that blood can't. It finds its way into the disks between the vertebrae of our spine. It is lymph fluid that provides them with their nutrients. The disks are those marvelous shock absorbers that help cushion our walk and allow flexibility in our back. In addition, lymph fluid carries away debris from between the cells. On its way through its channels, it passes through lymph nodes, where special Pac-Man-like cells gobble up any harmful bacteria, rendering them impotent. The debris carried away is eventually dumped into the blood circulation, where it is then filtered and processed by the liver, kidneys, and other organs of elimination.

Lymph nodes can become enlarged from an overload of bacteria, which occurs with certain types of infection. We usually refer to these enlarged lymph nodes as "swollen glands." Swollen glands are generally evidenced in the neck, in the armpits, and in the groin. Lymph nodes are concentrated in these areas because these are the areas where major movement takes place. These are where one large body part joins with another. Lymph fluid, you see, has no pump, no heart like the blood has to circulate it. It depends upon exercise and muscle movement to squeeze the nodes and thus propel it through the system. People who exercise a lot usually have a better working lymph system than do couch potatoes. Fitness is better than flab. Good lymphatic circulation is one major reason exercise is important. When you move your joints, you promote better lymphatic circulation. It is better to wear out than rust out.

Some people are inherently weak in the lymphatic department and display heavy congestion. They hold water in their tissues easily and may exhibit a slight puffiness of their face, hands, and feet. They may also gain weight easily and lose it only with difficulty. Most of their weight gain is associated with retention of this excess water. You should look for evidence of both chronic and acute congestion of the lymph nodes when examining an iris. When the lymph-congestion sign is not evident, it indicates a well-functioning lymph system that has little or no congestive problems. When it is present, lymph-node congestion usually appears in or near zones 5 and 6. Remember the iris zones? Lymph-node congestion is not always confined within the borders of these zones, but the zones are useful as a guide to approximate location.

Chronic lymph-node congestion appears as an off-white or slightly yellow coloration in discrete, almost cottony appearing puffs. In brown irides, it appears more yellowish than it does in blue irides. You may see one, two, or more of these patches. Sometimes a string of patches appears around the iris. (See Figure 6.4.) When this string appears, it can resemble beads, which is why the name "lymphatic rosary" was coined. A lymphatic rosary indicates heavy lymph congestion. If the congestion appears very white in certain areas, it signals acuteness. People with inherited tendencies toward lymphatic congestion, as displayed in the iris, will find it difficult, if not impossible, to do away with this iris sign.

The skin is the last of the five main elimination organs we will consider. It is one of the most important, even though most laymen do not generally think of it as an organ at all.

The average person eliminates about two pounds of waste material daily through the pores of his skin. People who engage in vigorous physical activity eliminate an even greater amount. We cannot live for more than a few hours if our skin elimination is severely curtailed. A burn victim who has had over 50 percent of his skin function destroyed has a lowered chance for survival. In addition to the risk of infection of his skin, his kidneys are placed under a terrific load because of the loss of elimination assistance by the skin. His kidneys now have the added burden of removing the uric-acid waste products that his skin normally eliminates. Burn victims frequently die from uremic poisoning, which is caused by a high concentration of uric acid in the blood. Uric acid is a normal end-product of metabolism, but it is toxic and must be continuously removed. Because the skin functions much the same as the kidneys do in removing these wastes, I like to call the skin our "third kidney."

Skin elimination is facilitated by exposing the skin to air and sunshine. But, however wonderful going around in the buff may be for better skin elimination, it is usually frowned upon by society. Thankfully, loose-fitting clothes and naturally absorbent fibers can help. So can wearing a minimum of clothes when the event and climate permit.

Poor skin elimination is evidenced in the iris by a darkened area in zone 7, the outermost zone on the chart. The darkened area will often extend a distance beyond this, into zone 6 and even zone 5. This dark area is called a "scurf rim." (See Figure

6.5.) The darker and wider the scurf rim is, the greater is the skin-elimination problem.

Nearly all irides reveal some degree of diminished skin function. However, it is most evident in people who dwell in cold climates and wear heavy clothing. Look for the scurf rim to be the heaviest from the 7:00 to 10:00 position and from 2:00 to 5:00. These represent the areas usually covered by clothing.

Look for a scurf rim in every iris you examine. You will seldom be disappointed. The greatest scurf rims I have ever seen were in the irides of nuns who were wearing the dark, tight-fitting habits of years past that did not allow the skin to breathe as it should. In recent years, most of these nuns have "kicked" their old habits and have blessed their skin elimination in the process.

The five main elimination channels are five extremely important systems to the body in general. This is because proper elimination is vital to good health. You can't have a good life with a poorly functioning, dirty interior. Look to the elimination channels—especially the bowel—first and you will never go wrong.

7.

The Rest of the Body Shows and Tells

The body's five main elimination channels are the most important keys to the door of good health, as we just discussed in Chapter 6, but there are several more locks that we must open before attaining our goal. Each of these additional keys, which we will discuss in this chapter, is important in its own right, performing specific functions for an individualized purpose. So, let's continue our peek at iridology in action and examine the brain areas, spine, glands, and circulatory system. We'll backtrack to the middle of the iris chart and start with the brain areas.

THE BRAIN AREAS

The brain areas are the most fascinating areas of the chart while at the same time the least understood. They are interesting from the standpoint that the brain is the master control for the entire body. This marvelous bioelectric computer has nearly incomprehensible limits, perhaps even no limits. So vast and complex is the brain that even the collective information gathered by modern man pertaining to its function is but minuscule compared with what has yet to be learned. No one dares even guess the outer limits of brain potential. It is widely accepted that the average person uses less than 10 percent of his brain potential. Some believe it's much less. The most powerful computers yet devised fall pitifully short of beginning to mimic true brain capability. And to top it all off, this vast biocomputing power is tucked neatly into a handsome, protective carrying case and balanced on top of your neck.

The brain, being what it is, does not readily lend itself to the exploration of its function or even of its anatomy. The gross anatomical examination of the brain of a deceased person doesn't reveal a great deal about function. Unlike a knee joint, which can be passively articulated even in death, the brain loses its entire ability to function upon the demise of its owner. In fact, the current criterion for death is the lack of any detectable brain activity. Since society frowns upon doing much in the way of experimentation with living brains (to say nothing of the feelings of those being experimented upon!), we know painfully little about the brain. In addition, when the brain is alive and working, it is a terribly subjective piece of equipment. This makes it very different from other anatomical parts. It seldom operates consistently from one person to another. In fact, it is not to be second-guessed even in the same person.

I hope I have made the point that it's more than a little difficult to obtain very much reliable or consistent information about the function of that maze of neurons above your shoulders known as the "brain." Recently, however, researchers utilizing the new technology of magnetic resonance imaging (MRI) have been able to learn some exciting new things about the living brain.

An illustration of how little we know about the brain concerns the function of memory, which we now know does not reside within the physical brain. We have been taught to think of the brain as a large computer and so we often think of memory as being contained in a memory bank, a physical storage space that contains "files" to be accessed at will. This technological-based thinking reveals our human orientation to time and space. However, scientists recently found that thoughts do not require a spatial domain for storage. Thought is not physical and thus requires no room. Our physical brain cells seem to provide merely the necessary bioelectrical means for recall, not storage space. We don't know where, if anywhere, memory is stored. However, it does not appear to be within the brain.

Here's something else to exercise your neurons. There are several people in the world—at present, about five or six—who demonstrate almost no brain at all. These people were discovered quite by accident when they were examined with MRI equipment. Very little brain matter was revealed within each one's skull. Nearly all of the small amount of brain material that was visualized was concentrated near the perimeter of the head, against the skull, as if deposited there by centrifugal force, like clothes clinging to the side of a washing machine after they have spun dry. The center of each person's head was, amazingly, quite hollow. Scientists are completely baffled by this odd situation. What's even more amazing is that none of these people are of diminished intelligence. In fact, some of them are above average. Nor do they have any other dysfunction that would suggest their unusual cerebral anatomy. One can only guess how many other people there are in the world with a similar situation.

We would do well to ponder the brain's relation to thought and cognitive function. This is definitely something for us all to think about. So, perhaps the stage has now been set for considering the brain areas listed on the iris chart.

On the iris chart, the brain areas collectively take up more space than any other organ. They are located between the 11:00 and 1:00 positions, with the animation life area specifically located at high noon. Of importance to iridologists is the observation that when tissue integrity is compromised in the animation life area, the person will frequently complain of, or at least admit to, chronic fatigue. When this is evident in both irides, the person nearly always complains that he is tired and lacking in stamina. Even with the other organs and systems possessing a relatively high degree of tissue integrity, if this little area at 12:00 is found wanting, there is usually a diminished energy level. I personally feel that all nerve energy enters the body through this particular brain area and is distributed from here to the autonomic nerve wreath and then to the entire body. My theory may provoke controversy, but it is an observation gained from many years in the practice of iridology.

There are iris signs other than those indicating inherent weakness and level of tissue integrity that can have a potent effect on the brain areas, especially on the animation life area. These signs are not depicted on the iris chart. Specifically, I am referring to the signs of brain anemia (anemia in extremities), the arcus senilis, and the cholesterol ring. We can also include the indicator of poor circulation, which, unlike the others, is represented on the iris chart as a ringed area bordering the skin area. All of these signs are related to circulation.

It is not difficult to make the connection between diminished circulation to the brain and compromised brain function. The presence of one or more of these iris signs, particularly anemia in extremities and the arcus senilis, is a good indicator of some degree of diminished brain function. Their presence affects the animation life area perhaps more than any other sign does, with the person experiencing fatigue and quickly running out of energy.

A person can inherit a weakness of the tissues in the animation life area as well as he can anywhere else. I believe that an inherent weakness in this area can be the reason some people lack stamina and energy all their life—even as children—tiring easily and requiring more rest and relaxation than others. Of course, we must keep in mind that this is but one area on the chart that may contribute to such an enervated condition.

Perhaps you have noticed that the animation life area is highlighted on the iris chart with a heavy outline. Notice, too, that it extends a little outside the chart circumference. There are several other areas that also extend just beyond the chart circumference. These are the areas that the iridologist considers first. Some of the areas gained their importance because they are major organs of elimination. They serve in one way or another to aid the body in ridding itself of toxic waste materials. The rest are important because they are essential in some other aspect of body function and are commonly the sites of inherent weakness. You can count on visualizing problems in these areas in the irides of people who have numerous or serious health complaints. Findings indicate that if we give priority to these highlighted areas, taking care to enhance tissue integrity there as quickly as possible, the whole body will usually respond with a greater sense of well-being.

In addition to the animation life area, the heavily outlined areas include the pineal gland, pituitary gland, heart, solar plexus, lungs and bronchi, prostate/uterus, penis/vagina, anus and rectum, kidneys and adrenals, ovaries/testes, spleen, appendix, liver and gall bladder, pancreas, and pleura and thorax areas. Notice also that the brain areas are collectively bounded by a heavy outline at 11:00 and 1:00.

Please call to mind again the segment of Hering's Law that states that all healing takes place *from the head down.* All healing begins in the mind and brain. Although we know very little about the brain area's specific iris signs, which are sometimes referred to as "brain flares," the lesions are nonetheless thought to be of considerable importance.

Another brain area that is individually highlighted is the medulla. The medulla is a part of the brain stem, which is that portion of the brain extending downward and eventuating in the spinal cord. It is the primitive brain in many lower animals. In man's evolutionary development, it is much older than the higher brain centers, anatomically located above it. The medulla is also known to iridologists as the "chest-brain." This is because it normally controls our breathing rate. We don't have to think about when to breathe. Even when unconscious, we normally maintain our breathing. Iridologists have observed that when there is an inherited weakness displayed in the medulla area, the lungs are often compromised in their function. This is because the developing lungs do not receive as strong a nerve impulse from the medulla as they should.

We can do deep-breathing exercises, especially one known as "sniff breathing," to increase our vital lung capacity. Sniff breathing is a technique developed and taught by the late Thomas Gaines. He taught it to the New York City Police Department. Sniff breathing, executed while walking briskly, consists of taking a series of short and forceful inhalations in time with your steps until your lungs are completely filled. With your lungs fully expanded, you hold your breath for a few seconds or a couple of steps. You then forcefully expel it in a single, rapid exhalation. Vital lung capacity is the volume of air we breathe in during inhalation. Regularly practicing sniff breathing increases this volume. This aids in the oxygenation of the blood, which translates directly into greater energy and vitality.

When the medulla is weak, we have a lowered vital capacity.

The lungs fail to develop as they should, and the chest does not expand as much as it ought to due to the shallow breathing. This is why we call the medulla the "chest-brain." Conversely, an inherently strong tissue integrity in the medulla area usually results in automatic deeper breathing, an increased vital capacity in the lungs, and an expanded chest cavity. When you observe the medulla area in the iris, you should also check the lung and bronchial areas for weakness. When a weakness is visualized in the medulla area, a corresponding weakness is frequently found in the lung or bronchials.

Besides controlling the breathing rate, the medulla also exercises a measure of control over the heart rate. Oxygenation of the blood indirectly affects heart rate, too. Other parameters remaining unchanged, tissues supplied with well-oxygenated blood cause the heart rate to be reduced. This makes less work for the heart. At every turn, we are reminded of the interdependency of all organs.

In my large and complete iridology textbook for serious students and practitioners of the healing arts, I go into each brain area in depth. There has been considerable information gathered through observation of the brain areas, but much is still sketchy and unproven. Dr. Kritzer devoted a lifetime to iridology and felt he had located the brain area associated with epilepsy. He called this area the "epileptic center." I carried this name on my early iris charts, but I have since changed it to "equilibrium dizziness center" because I now associate this area with some conditions other than epilepsy. Once again, I would like to stress that we need to learn a lot more about these brain areas represented on the iris chart. If you would like additional information about them or about brain function, please refer to my aforementioned text, *Iridology: The Science and Practice in the Healing Arts, Volume II.*

Just above the brain areas and outside the periphery of the chart are printed the functions of the brain area directly below. These functions are in mirror-image—reversed—in the left and right irides. Current thought holds that the brain areas in the left iris from 12:00 to 1:00 are more closely associated with the physiological, cerebellar, and sensory functions of the brain than are those areas from 11:00 to 12:00, which are more attuned to the psychological, cerebral, and motor functions.

I should mention that the brain areas contain two glands: the pineal gland, designated "p" on the iris chart, and the pituitary gland, designated "pit. g." These glands are placed in the brain areas because anatomically, they reside within the brain.

With regard to the brain areas, it is ironic and indeed unfortunate that the organ occupying the largest area on the iris chart and responsible for control of the entire body is the one we know the least about. The brain, an organ weighing a mere two-and-a-half pounds yet controlling nearly everything, is indeed a marvel. As you examine the brain areas, look for healing lines in addition to inherent weaknesses and lesions. It is interesting to note that for many years, scientists claimed that certain types of nerve tissue did not regenerate, but this has been called into question in recent studies. Even though it is accepted that nerve tissue is very slow to heal—much slower than almost any other tissue—it is no longer safe to say that certain nerve tissue does not regenerate at all. You can find healing signs in the brain areas, too. Look for them.

THE SPINE

In the United States alone, 75 million people have back problems. There are over 7 million new victims each year. Some 5 million of these are partly disabled and 2 million are totally disabled. Back problems are the second leading cause of hospitalization (remember, digestive disorders are number one). There are 93 million workdays lost each year due to back problems and much of this lost work time is due to injury.

Injuries to the spine, which is labelled "back" on the iris chart, rank as the number-one injury in the workplace. Americans spend $5 billion each year on back injuries. This is in addition to the $12–20 billion paid out by insurance companies for disability claims, lawsuits, and settlements. Nearly everyone at some time experiences the agonizing discomfort of back pain, which is reason enough to look to the iris and see what can be learned.

It was old Hippocrates, the father of medicine, who reminded us that in all illness, we should look to the spine as well as to the bowel. The profession of chiropractic, the second largest healing profession in the United States and boasting the largest group of drugless healers, has built its practice around the spine being the backbone of good health. The success of this healing art is due directly to the anatomical fact that the nerves emanating from between the spinal vertebrae serve nearly all the areas of the body. Not only do these spinal nerves provide for energy flow outward from the brain, they also transmit information received from the tissues and organs back to the brain for processing. The brain can then evaluate this neurological data and make the necessary adjustments to maintain equilibrium in the system.

Proper nerve-energy flow to the organs and tissues promotes and sustains tissue integrity. Faults in the delivery of this nerve energy result directly in a compromise of tissue integrity. As we have seen, a compromised or diminished tissue integrity translates directly into altered function. Altered function then produces symptoms. Frequently, specifically directed spinal adjustment by the skilled hands of a chiropractor is most beneficial in restoring compromised nerve-energy flow. This is a fact confirmed daily by the many satisfied patients in every chiropractic office in the land.

In addition to its neurological component, the spine is a biomechanical structural support. It is a part of what is known as the "axial skeleton." In other words, it serves as a strong yet flexible pillar that supports all the structures above the pelvic base and enables us to walk upright as well as to flex in every direction.

All health-care practitioners would be enlightened to know what the iris can reveal about this marvelous organ. Chiropractors in particular could use iris analysis to collect data concerning the inherent weaknesses in a spine. Weaknesses contribute in no small way to a person's need for chiropractic care and to an understanding of how he should order his lifestyle, work, and nutrition to avoid, or at least minimize, spinal problems.

The spine is commonly divided into four sections. At the top is the cervical spine, so named because "cervices" is Latin for "neck." Next is the thoracic spine, named because of its association with the thorax, or chest. Then comes the lumbar spine, which is the area most people associate with a backache.

It is often referred to as the "low back." These three parts—the cervical, thoracic, and lumbar spine—all joined together, sit atop a large, triangular, wedge-shaped bone called the "sacrum." The sacrum is actually part of the pelvic structure but is often thought of as part of the spine. It has, however, an intimate relationship with the mechanics of the lower back and is the platform, or base, upon which the spine rests.

The iris chart graphically depicts the spine as divided into four sections roughly corresponding to the cervical, thoracic, lumbar, and sacral portions. These are found in the left iris between the 7:20 and 8:25 positions, and as a mirror image in the right iris between 3:35 and 4:40. Please note that the sacrum is not labelled on the chart and that the other areas are simply referred to as the "upper," "middle," and "lower" back.

The iris chart does not pretend to be accurate enough to place an iris sign at a particular vertebral level or segment. Given the present stage of chart development, it is satisfactory to generally locate any iris sign in the upper, middle, or lower back, with the unlabelled sacrum included in the lower back area.

We usually think of tissue as being soft and fleshy, but the cells that make up the human organism are diverse indeed. Mature bone cells look quite different under a microscope than do other types of cells, but they, too, are alive and have their special activity. For instance, we don't often think of blood as a tissue, but it is classified as such. Tissues can range from liquid to hard, compact bone. No matter what its form, each cell composing a tissue has its individual level of integrity. Bone cells with a decreased integrity are weak and thus subject to infection, disease, and fracture.

A most important concept to understand is that when we look in the iris at the back areas, we should not confine our thoughts to bone. The spine has many muscles attached to it. It also has ligamentous tissue, nerve tissue, lymphatic tissue, and countless small blood vessels. Don't let the graphic depiction of the bony spine on the iris chart lead you to exclude its attached, and closely allied, soft tissue structures. The great majority of back pain is associated not so much with the hard, bony structure as it is with the muscles and ligaments attached to it or functionally associated with it.

A one-sided inherent weakness in the spine is frequently associated with an abnormal curvature of the back, known as "scoliosis." Look for weaknesses in the irides of people who have moderate to severe spinal curvatures. An inherent weakness can also make someone susceptible to strains, sprains, and recurring back injury. Chiropractors, orthopedists, osteopaths, naprapaths, masseurs, and other practitioners who witness a great many back problems in their daily practice could benefit by looking to the iris. Inherent weakness in the back areas predisposes a person to recurring subluxations as weak ligaments fail to limit a joint to its normal range of motion. Often, iris signs in the spinal areas can help explain to both doctor and questioning patient why there is a propensity for injury or recurrent subluxation in a particular area. Chiropractors usually find that barring traumatic injury, a person who is unable to hold his adjustment displays an inherent weakness in the corresponding back area in the iris.

In your analysis of the iris, note any weaknesses in the back. You may want to try confirming your observations by asking your subject if he ever had any spinal trouble and specifically where the trouble was. Inherent weakness in the back is no different than a similar weakness elsewhere. There can be various types of lesions and also healing lines. Once again, we should remember to think in terms of tissue integrity. Lesions indicative of inherent weakness can appear anywhere in the back areas and are not confined to the graphic representation of the spine on the iris chart. For example, you can find a weakness in zone 4 or 5 in the upper back area. The lesion or weakness does not need to be confined to zone 3 to be associated with the upper back. This is true for all the divisions of the back. Iridology should be an enlightening experience and a joy to practice. Have fun!

OUR GLANDULAR POWERHOUSE

Many years ago, when I visited San Francisco, I took a trip to the powerhouse for the famous cable cars of that city. There I saw some of the most powerful electric motors I'd ever seen. These motors slowly turned the large wheels that carried the endless loop of cable running under the city streets to which the cable cars, overflowing with riders, would attach themselves. In this manner, the cars could be drawn up or restrained while ascending and descending the steep hills of that unique and beautiful city. The glands of the body may be small in size, but like the cable-car motors, they are very powerful. They control our thinking, our desires, our actions, and even our strength and willpower. Our glands enable us to climb up the emotional hills of life and be let safely down the steep descents. There isn't anything about us they don't influence. They determine our degree of masculinity and femininity, our body build, our emotions, and even our thoughts. We cannot live without them.

Glands are the chemical laboratories where hormones and enzymes are made. Hormones are extremely powerful even in very minute amounts and the body responds almost instantly to changes in their concentration in the blood. Glands are responsible for growth and development, as well as for aging. Glandular function drops off about 20 percent near the age of forty and then continues to slowly diminish thereafter. We feel, and are, as young as our glandular functions. This is why people say that you are as young as you feel. I have said in my lectures that we are as young as our glands. Our glands determine if we feel young in our golden years or old before our time.

The iris chart illustrates quite a number of glands, from the Peyer's patches and pea-sized pineal gland, labelled "pey. pat." and "p," respectively, to the large, dual-lobed, and powerful thyroid gland. Glands are so complex in their function that the story of even one gland would be a book in itself. There are basically two major classifications of glands: glands with ducts and glands without ducts. Those having ducts, which carry the glandular secretions to a particular point, have a more localized effect. The ductless glands, on the other hand, release their secretions directly into the bloodstream. These latter glands are known as the endocrine glands. They elicit extremely fast, system-wide responses.

Think of the time it would take the adrenal glands to respond if you unexpectedly met a bear in the woods. The response time would be so short that it would be considered immediate. Other glands are just as powerful but much slower. An example of these is the pituitary gland, labelled "pit. g." on the chart, which controls our size and rate of growth. The pituitary gland is also known as the "master gland" because it sends out hormones to specifically influence and control other glands. Glands exercise control, and are themselves controlled, by elaborate and delicately balanced biochemical feedback pathways.

The pancreas, "pan." on the iris chart, is a gland that secretes enzymes necessary for digestion. It also produces insulin to metabolize sugar. It is impossible to maintain life without pancreatic function. Sugar diabetes is frequently a result of dysfunction in a part of this gland. The pancreas is represented on the chart for the right iris, near the autonomic nerve wreath, at the 7:00 position. Being a right-hand organ, it is not represented in the left iris.

Peyer's patches are little patches of lymph-like glands in the small intestine that are mysterious in their function. Lesions there are often associated with fevers, especially typhoid fever. Damage to these lymphoid patches and a history of fevers are sometimes associated with abnormal weight gain or the inability to lose weight and keep it off. Look for the Peyer's patches in the small-intestine area of both irides. Again, they are depicted on the chart by a cluster of small dots labelled "pey. pat."

The thyroid gland regulates our metabolic rate, which is the speed of our body's internal clock. A sluggish thyroid gland may be associated with obesity, mental dullness, feelings of coldness, and a lack of ambition, whereas an overactive thyroid can cause the opposite reactions. The thyroid gland is positioned at the midline of the body and has a right and a left lobe. Quite often, iridologists find that one lobe is underactive while the other lobe is overactive to compensate. Laboratory thyroid tests using the blood generally show nothing unusual in these cases, but the imbalance, found through iris analysis, can cause problems. The thyroid gland is found at 9:30 on the left chart and in the mirror-image location on the right.

The label "p.t." on the iris chart stands for "parathyroid." "Para" is Greek for "around" or "about," and the parathyroid glands are around, or about, the thyroid gland. These glands help control the calcium reserves in the body. They are a kind of balance to the functions of the thyroid gland. Abnormalities in parathyroid function can cause someone to be susceptible to the formation of kidney stones. This is because the parathyroid glands help control the body's calcium and lime salts, which can form these stones. The parathyroid glands are located on the iris chart in the center of the bronchus area, at the nerve wreath.

The thymus gland, which is not illustrated on some iris charts, is marked "thy" on the Jensen chart. In the body, it is located in the upper chest cavity, above and in front of the heart. It is large in children but normally shrinks in size with age so that it is very small at maturity. It is associated with the production of T-cells, which are special cells of the immune system that form a strong line of defense against disease. T-cell-destruction is one factor associated with the disease of AIDS. Removal of the thymus gland in childhood stimulates gonadal development. In contrast, an overactive thymus retards the development of strong sexual differentiation. The thymus gland is located on the Jensen chart for the left iris, at the wreath, immediately below the heart.

The little pineal gland is located in the brain. Its function has long been debated. Some people say that it is a rudimentary third eye and is sensitive to light. A lot of mystery surrounds this controversial little gland, which is about the size of a pea. Several experts believe it has a balancing effect against the action of light upon the pigment of the skin, acting in conjunction with the adrenal glands in regulating skin pigmentation. The pineal is also connected with sexual and mental attainments, as well as with the development of the spiritual side of life. As mentioned, the pineal gland is labelled with a "p" and located at 11:10 on the left chart and 12:50 on the right chart.

Most people don't realize that the appendix is a gland. It is composed of lymph-like tissue and its function is to secrete lubricants to "oil" the ileo-cecal valve, which is the important valve at the juncture of the small and large intestines. I already mentioned that the function of the ileo-cecal valve is to keep colon contents from backing up into the small intestine. Because of this, contrary to the opinion of some, the appendix is not a useless appendage. People who have had their appendix removed are susceptible to ileo-cecal-valve dysfunction. In reality, inflammation of the appendix seldom necessitates surgery if proper, conservative care is instituted without delay. The appendix can be found at the 6:30 position on the right iris chart and is labelled "append."

The liver is also not commonly considered a gland, but it does produce bile, which is a secretion that is concentrated and stored in the gall bladder. Bile is one of the most noxious substances produced in the body. It is very bitter and toxic. It is carried from the gall bladder through a duct into the intestine, where it stimulates peristalsis to help move the bowel. Bile also helps to emulsify fats in the diet, which is necessary for their proper absorption. If the bile duct is obstructed, digestive troubles result immediately, followed by the development of yellow skin (jaundice). Incidentally, before the skin changes color, the sclera (white) of the eye becomes yellow. This situation must be corrected quickly because of the toxic nature of bile.

The kidneys, like the appendix and liver, are also not usually thought of as glands, but they, too, produce glandular-like substances. You can begin to see that if the glands are broadly defined, quite a number of organs can be so labelled.

The ovaries in the female and testes in the male are also glands. Each has its particular secretion for the reproduction of life. In addition, both these glands secrete hormones that are needed by, and present in, both sexes: females have some male hormones and males have some female hormones. The ovaries in the female produce hormones that can result, when unbalanced, in a litany of complaints every month as the menstrual cycle dips and peaks. It is not uncommon for some women to suffer terribly due to a minor, yet very troublesome, glandular imbalance.

The prostate gland in the male is associated with the secretion and storage of seminal fluid. Disturbances in this gland are common in advancing years and can cause irritability, depression, and even suicidal tendencies. Men can have their glandular troubles, too! On the chart, the prostate gland is labelled "pro." and shares the same location as the uterus ("ut.") in the female. Truly, all our glands powerfully influence our life. Human beings display a wondrous and most delicate balance of a vast array of enzymes and hormones. To disturb this balance, even slightly, can be very dangerous.

When you observe the iris and see inherent weaknesses or other lesions in the glands, you must be very careful about what you conclude. Because of glandular interaction, a weakness in one gland can cause compensations in other glands. Dual glands (such as the kidneys and adrenals) have lots of reserve power. A weakness in one side, or even removal, may not produce any symptoms.

Glandular evaluation utilizing iris analysis is a highly developed art. Look for an inherent weakness in the glands, as well as for signs of overactivity. Try to relate what you see to any complaints the patient may have. This is how to learn. But please remember that while the glands can cause very powerful reactions, so can your comments about them. My son David had an expression as a boy: "Use your carefulness." That expression certainly applies when evaluating the glands.

THE CIRCULATORY INDICATORS

There are four iris signs that are linked by a common thread. They are the arcus senilis, the anemia in extremities sign, the cholesterol ring (also called the "sodium ring"), and finally, the circulatory ring. Of these four, only the last one is labelled on the iris chart. It is part of the lymphatic and circulatory systems ring comprising zone 6. The others are not labelled because doing so would create confusion. When present, they can overlay, and sometimes totally obscure, some of the other labelled areas. Besides, they do not represent any normal anatomical structure as do nearly all the other labelled sections of the chart.

We shall consider the four circulatory indicators in the order listed. The first is the arcus senilis. Translated literally, the name of this sign means "arc of old age." It is so called because it appears in the shape of an arc, or crescent. (See Figure 6.6 in Chapter 6.) Also, it is more commonly found in the elderly than in the young.

The arcus senilis appears in zone 7 in the brain areas and, with increased severity, can extend down to overlay zones 5 and 6. It is a translucent, or semitransparent, bluish-gray veil that seems to be continuous with the sclera. It looks almost as if the sclera is trying to come up over the iris and, in so doing, obliterates the defined iris margin. When heavier and more extensive, it can cover a significant portion of the brain areas.

Despite its name, the arcus senilis sign is not limited to the elderly. Sometimes it is visualized in younger people as well. It always indicates diminished oxygenation to the representative areas it covers. Because the arcus senilis does not represent a specific organ or tissue, it is not represented on the iris chart.

The hands and feet are the portions of the body that are the farthest removed from the heart. This is why the legs, feet, forearms, and hands are referred to as the "extremities." Blood has to be pumped quite a distance to reach these extreme points, and then it must return, usually uphill, against the force of gravity.

You could also think of the brain as a sort of extremity. It sits at the extreme top of the axial skeleton, or spinal column. Even though, physically, it is not very far removed from the heart, it requires a constant and copious flow of oxygenated blood to perform its functions. Even a mild, temporary reduction in the flow of blood to the brain will result in a feeling of wooziness, a feeling of losing it, and even fainting. Mild, chronic restrictions of blood flow will result in forgetfulness and fuzzy thinking. At normal body temperature, seriously decreased circulation to the brain for more than four minutes can result in permanent brain damage. As you can see, the presence of an arcus senilis is synonymous with brain anemia, or hypoxia, which is a lack of adequate oxygenation of the brain tissues.

When the arcus senilis sign appears in the lower extremities area, iridologists refer to it as "anemia in extremities." (See Figure 6.7 in Chapter 6.) It simply is manifest in another location in the iris. Instead of, or in addition to, appearing in the upper portion of the iris, the anemia in extremities sign appears at the bottom. Just as the arcus senilis sign indicates poor circulation to the brain areas, the anemia in extremities sign testifies to poor circulation in the legs.

The anemia in extremities and arcus senilis signs often occur together. People with anemia in extremities have the usual problems that come with poor circulation in the legs and feet: cold feet, aching and tired legs, and other conditions associated with arterial and venous congestive states. Few people, even the relatively young, have perfect circulation to the brain and extremities. The early traces of an arcus senilis or anemia in extremities sign can frequently be found in the iris.

The next circulatory indicator we will consider is the cholesterol ring. Sometimes called the "sodium ring," it is found in the same areas as the arcus senilis and anemia in extremities signs. However, unlike the first two signs, the cholesterol ring is milky white in appearance and always opaque, obscuring totally any iris structure it covers. (See Figure 6.8 in Chapter 6.) Also, it does not appear to be continuous with the sclera and it may manifest as a complete ring. Those with heavy inorganic-sodium intake over an extended period may exhibit a dense, opaque, milky ring in zones 6 and 7. Such a ring is sometimes seen in a person who has spent much of his life at sea or near the ocean, eating salt foods and breathing salt air.

Inorganic sodium—sodium that does not come into the body through plants and animals in the diet—acts as a hardener in the body. It hardens the arteries and joints. A heavy sodium ring in the iris is also known as a cholesterol ring because elevated cholesterol deposits in the arteries have been found to coincide with the sign's appearance in the iris. In fact, a recent article in *Reader's Digest* said, "Results of a new study, published in the *Journal of the American Optometric Association*, show that, regardless of age, patients with the white ring—known as the corneal arcus—had higher blood-cholesterol levels and thus a greater risk of heart disease. Previously the ring was considered a normal part of aging."

Cholesterol can accumulate on arterial walls in the form of fatty plaques that restrict normal blood flow. When blood flow is restricted, it can cause high blood pressure as the heart seeks to maintain blood-flow volume. As the arterial walls harden from the long-term intake of inorganic sodium, they lose their elasticity, which, in turn, can cause a rise in the diastolic blood pressure, the pressure when our heart is at rest between beats. For many years, I, as well as other iridologists, have associated the white arc in the iris with elevated cholesterol. I have been referring to it in my books as the "cholesterol ring." Iridology has been, and still is, ahead of its time. Ideas ahead of their time are usually ridiculed or ignored. However, medical science will eventually catch up as iris sign by iris sign, the validity of iridology is confirmed.

The white appearance of the cholesterol ring is what I also call "calcium out of solution." I believe that inorganic sodium causes calcium to be less soluble and that undissolved calcium then settles in tissues in which it normally would not settle. It can slowly build up in the lens of the eye and eventually create cataracts. It can also settle in the joints and is associated with the calcium deposits seen on x-ray in cases of arthritis. This calcium settlement creates a hardness, a stiffness. It can cause the joints to stiffen. It can harden the arteries, which then lose their elasticity. When this happens, the first sign is often an elevated blood pressure, and later, clogging of the arteries. I believe inorganic elements in the body can cause a lot of trouble as they accumulate.

Many other things can also interfere with circulation. Inorganic mineral salts besides sodium—such as the aluminum in baking powder, mercury salts, inorganic mineral salts dissolved in hard water, and even the salt used to soften water in water-softening units—can be associated with problems. Add to this the hardened fats from fried foods and the various synthetic products created when natural fats are unnaturally hydrogenated by food manufacturers. Lecithin, a naturally occurring fat in some foods and in all foods containing cholesterol, is chemically changed when exposed to temperatures above the boiling point (212°F.). Since lecithin serves to emulsify cholesterol, its destruction by too much heat can cause a cholesterol buildup in the body. The intake of cholesterol without the emulsifying action of lecithin can dangerously raise the cholesterol level of the blood. Cholesterol itself is not a villain in food. How we process and cook foods are the problems. It is wise to remember that nature's creations are perfect. *Man*handled food is the problem.

Manhandled food is also associated with many of society's ills and chronic diseases. Rheumatism, arthritis, osteoporosis, cataracts, heart troubles, and circulatory degenerative diseases—to name but a few—all have strong links to improper nutrition. As time passes, researchers are finding that chronic degenerative diseases have greater associations with nutrition than they previously thought possible. We can see the effects of improper nutrition in the iris.

The last of the circulatory indicators we will examine is the circulatory ring. I mentioned the circulatory ring earlier, along with the fact that it is supposed to appear in zone 6 of the iris chart. However, like the lymphatic rosary and lymph-congestive conditions, also depicted in zone 6, it does not confine itself within the neat, stylized boundary on the chart. Whereas lymphatic congestion is usually evidenced more toward the pupil side of the zone, in practice, the circulatory ring is visualized on the very periphery of the iris. Thus, the circulatory ring is seen on the peripheral side of zone 7, the skin zone. In cases of venous congestion, it appears as a bluish-purple ring. (See Figure 6.9 in Chapter 6.) Venous congestion, of course, is a circulatory condition. I think immediately of varicose veins when I see this indicator. Varicosities result from increased pressures due to the poor venous return of blood, which, when combined with dysfunction of the little check valves, causes distention of the thin walls of the involved veins.

Look for the circulatory indicators we just discussed in every iris you examine. They are more common than you might think. When you see any of these signs, you will know that the owner has, or is on his way to developing, a circulatory condition. And after observing a number of irides, you will understand why circulatory disease is the number-one killer of Americans.

You now have an expanding list of signs to look for in the iris. Please remember to *ask* the people you examine if they are having any difficulty with the problems you see in their irides. *Ask;* don't tell. Be mindful of who you are. If you are not a doctor with diagnostic training and lots of experience, it is better to *ask* than to *tell*. Remember, even the well-trained diagnostician makes his share of mistakes. It is said that the fool is proud because he knows so much; the wise person is humble because he knows so little.

THE REST OF THE STORY

There are some areas on the iris chart that are less important than others. This is not to say, however, that they are insignificant. Obviously, there is no area of the body that is unrelated to the whole and unworthy of consideration. But to comment on each and every area on the chart is not my purpose. My purpose is to acquaint you enough with the art and science of iridology so that you have a good feeling for what it is and how it works. Toward this end, I have discussed the definition and philosophy of iris analysis, iris-chart development, major iris signs, and some basic observations. All the areas of the iris chart, however, need to be considered when performing an iris analysis. I would like to give an example of how to look at these other areas and make useful determinations that can affect a person's life and health. Sometimes a story is the best example.

Some years ago, a young lady complaining of lower back pain visited Dr. Bodeen. In the course of his routine examination of her, Dr. Bodeen analyzed her irides. Among several iris signs worthy of note was a major inherent weakness in the vocal cords/trachea area in both irides. Even though the young woman had never complained of any problem in her vocal-cords area, in the course of the history-taking conversation, she related that she was aspiring to sing professionally and was taking voice lessons. When Dr. Bodeen asked how she was coming along with her lessons, however, she said her teacher had told her she had a good voice but that it lacked stamina. The teacher didn't know if her voice would be able to hold up under the strain of constant practice and the demands of professional work.

Because of the iridology examination, Dr. Bodeen felt it was his duty to suggest to the young woman that pursuing a singing career might not be in her best interest due to the inherited weakness he observed in her vocal cords. Of course, there was no reason she could not continue to sing in a nonprofessional capacity, where she would not have the demands imposed by a career. Dr. Bodeen was gratified when the young woman subsequently thanked him for providing her with this information. She had come to realize that her voice was not one of her stronger assets and, as a result, changed careers. She is now happy and successful in an alternate vocation.

Not everyone utilizing iris analysis will have the chance to effect such a change in another person's life. This illustration merely points out the need to consider all areas and to analyze what a lesion observed in one particular area could mean to a person as a whole.

The mental and spiritual sides of an individual need to be considered as well as the physical side. Not a few people have a job that is taxing to their inherently weak areas. They would serve themselves better to learn of their weaknesses and take up work that is more suitable to their specific physical and mental makeup.

You should examine every area for inherent weakness, chronic and degenerate lesions, white fibers indicating acuteness, drug settlements, and healing lines. You should evaluate each iris sign for its impact on every other area. For instance, even though you do not visualize any lesions in the thigh/knee/foot area, you might find an anemia in extremities sign that impacts on the circulation to that area. You might not find any lesions in the mastoid area of the left iris, but perhaps you'll find a very dark, chronic bowel pocket at the splenic flexure just opposite the mastoid. This bowel pocket can reflexly influence the mastoid. There are many more relationships that you could and should consider to perform a competent iris analysis. I am only touching on what is a multitude of possible relationships.

What we have learned in this book is just a beginning. There are many other complex relationships in the iris. For example, chart areas that are 180 degrees opposite each other have a special relationship. In addition, those at 90-degree angles have a special relationship. Iridologists still need to do a good bit of research on these angular relationships.

Although iris analysis can stand alone as a valuable analytic tool, it is best utilized in conjunction with other examination procedures as part of a professional diagnostic workup. This is most important when symptoms or suspicions of an underlying disease process are present. Furthermore, no single examination procedure should be exclusively relied upon in making a definitive diagnosis. Diagnostic and analytic tools should, whenever possible, be combined to achieve the highest possible accuracy in an attempt to serve the best interests of the individual in need. The day will come when, in the evaluation of the integrity of an organ, we will see that we are looking at tissue response. We will find that this response is based upon the tissue's integrity, its degree of inherent and attained strength. In addition, I believe that the iris will someday teach us about the proper food chemistry needed for each organ to function at its highest possible level.

I hope that your interest in iridology will grow and that I have motivated you to further study this challenging and exciting field. I hope that you see the close association of iridology with nutrition, tissue integrity, and body chemistry. Iris analysis is an expanding and exciting science. I believe that we are witnessing only the beginning of what is possible. As I frequently comment in my lectures, I believe there is more to be revealed in the iris than man will ever know. This I firmly believe.

Conclusion

T his chapter is entitled "Conclusion," but that's really a misnomer. As just mentioned at the end of Chapter 7, iris analysis has barely finished cracking out of its shell. Let's finish our discussion now by examining where iridology stands in today's world and where it may someday lead.

IRIS ANALYSIS COMPLEMENTS ALL HEALING ARTS

No method of examination, analysis, or diagnosis can truly stand alone. In reality, it is at best only one part of what might be done to raise a person to optimum health. Responses in the form of treatment, therapy, education, and perhaps lifestyle changes must form major scenes in the health-care picture of the future. I can't think of any health profession that would not be substantially enhanced by the employment of iris analysis.

Iris analysis itself is best employed in conjunction with the drugless healing arts. Included in these drugless arts are chiropractic, naprapathy, naturopathy, homeopathy, acupuncture, nutrition, and massage, as well as many other disciplines. This is not to say, however, that iris analysis would not be a wonderful complement to orthodox, allopathic medicine. No responsible person would deny that there is opportunity for the employment of drugs and surgery, although most would agree that orthodox medicine suffers from frequent abuses. Rather than being looked upon as the treatment of choice by society, allopathic therapy might better be considered for emergency-care situations and for those times when the more-natural methods have failed. Even so, iridology could greatly aid the allopathic physician. Elective surgical cases could be influenced by an awareness of the inherent weaknesses and strengths of the patients. Allopaths should be eager to refer persons to drugless physicians when appropriate. Referral should be a two-way street, always keeping the thought of maximum benefit to the patient in mind.

A growing number of iridologists are health-care professionals who employ their particular speciality in treating patients. They use iris analysis as an adjunctive method to their regular examination. Like laypersons, they refer patients for appropriate medical care when indicated. It is always ethical and prudent, as well as legally mandated, for a practitioner, lay or professional, to refer an individual to those who can best render the appropriate care. Ethics dictate that the welfare of the client or patient be held above all other considerations.

The layperson will not be long engaged in the study of iridology before he absolutely and convincingly sees the benefit of iris analysis as a complement to the healing arts. I believe it will be the layperson, the educated health-care consumer, who will force good and lasting changes upon what has been an ultraconservative, politically corrupt, and moribund system. People of good will and conviction will welcome the day when all health-care providers will be free to work together toward the common goals of minimizing suffering and maximizing health.

THE NUTRITION CONNECTION

I have purposely confined this book to the *analysis* of the iris. I have not gone into the remedies, the treatments, or the many and varied therapies that may be used to relieve or correct the conditions observed in the iris. Since those who employ iris analysis are from varied disciplines in the healing arts, many different therapeutic regimens are selectively employed to give comfort and to promote the healing process.

It has been my experience that the greatest single therapeutic regimen one can employ is the art and science of nutrition. This is the premier health science. All other therapeutic applications depend, in the long run, on proper considerations of nutrition. Without wholesome nutrition, all treatments, therapies, and medicaments ultimately fail.

Chiropractic is a wonderful therapeutic discipline, but it can be enhanced greatly with nutrition. Likewise, homeopathy, as good as it is, can be augmented with nutrition. Traditional allopathic medicine, with its shameful historical neglect of nutritional science, is now beginning to awaken to the role that nutrition can play in the maintenance and restoration of health. There is no discipline anyone can name that would not be improved with the addition of nutritional therapy. In fact, no discipline can be effective without it.

I have long contended that all acquired disease is closely tied to improper nutrition. Medical science has found in recent years, and is continuing to increasingly discover, a nutritional relationship to diseases once thought to have little or no connection at all with diet. I have found, and can safely say, that nearly every disease is associated with a chemical nutritional deficiency.

Perhaps the closest that iris analysis is tied to any follow-up therapy, except perhaps in Germany, is with the science of nutrition. As the song goes, "Love and marriage go together like a horse and carriage." Nutrition and iris analysis also go together. Like the horse and carriage, they belong to one another. What the iridologist usually sees when he views the irides is a graphic depiction of the results of long-term nutritional deficiency. I have repeatedly stated, in my lectures and books, that I do not believe there is any disease that is not associated with a nutritional deficiency. In my many years of practice at my health ranches, I have found this to be true over and over again. Now, the reverse of this, I believe, is that no true healing can take place—and be visualized in the iris— without nutritional provisions first being implemented.

Both iridology and nutrition employ completely natural, noninvasive methods. Neither requires even a modest invasion of a person's physical privacy. Nor do they employ medications of any kind. It was Hippocrates, the father of medicine, who admonished, "Let food be your medicine and medicine your food." I have endeavored to be a follower of this noble and ancient physician all my professional life and I attribute my best work to his timeless maxim.

Most people think of nutrition and diet as concerning just food and drink. As I previously mentioned, it is much more. You may have a nice, fresh garden salad in your diet every day. That's wonderful! But what about a diet of friends? Friends influence health more than you may realize. How about a diet of music? Wouldn't you like to have music as part of your diet? What music would you select? Music is food every bit as much as carrots or a delicious health drink. Good music nourishes every cell of the body.

How about color? Yes, there is a diet of color. A person can get sick when surrounded with drab, dull colors. By the same token, he can be lifted out of the doldrums by a lively splash of color. Color is food. We are nourished by it. We can feel blue, be green with envy, feel in the pink, or be yellow with fear. Color-therapy techniques for healing are very controversial, but we will see them become more and more accepted as their efficacy is scientifically explored and validated in time to come.

What about thoughts? What a person finds himself thinking about is his food for thought. We all have a diet of thoughts. "Thoughts are things" is an expression. We can't do anything without the thought first being there. That's something to think about, isn't it? Through applied kinesiology techniques, we can easily demonstrate how a negative thought can immediately cause a temporary weakness in the muscles. Imagine what a steady diet of negative thoughts will do! Diet is also the air we breathe, the sights we see, the aromas we smell, and everything we touch. *Our diet is the sum total of our life experiences.* It is all that we take in and absorb, by whatever medium. Nutrition is how our life is nurtured, mentally, physically, and spiritually.

A diet of frustrating thoughts can result in nerve rings in your iris, the same way that a poor diet from the dinner table can produce ill effects on your stomach. A diet of certain colors can lead you to see red or fall into a black depression. A diet of inorganic crude minerals can leave a stain in your iris, not unlike the way a bad experience can leave a stain on your mind. The mind, although not physical, can be as sensitive as the skin. Have you ever been rubbed the wrong way? If not, maybe it's because you're thick skinned. Remember, a compliment is like unto a sweet parfait; derision, like a sour lemon. Be careful to what you expose yourself. Likewise, be mindful of what you give forth to others. I hope you can see from these illustrations that everything you think and do, everything you see and hear—all you come in contact with in your world—is just as much a part of your diet as is an apple or a pear, a salad or a glass of carrot juice. You make choices about your diet with your every thought. You may have the finest health food and have its value severely compromised by a diet of stressful living.

In a recent survey, the United States Food and Drug Administration (FDA) found that over 40 percent of the population tested was low on calcium. One reason for the survey was the alarming rise in osteoporosis in postmenopausal women. Osteoporosis is a loss of mineralization of the bones. It was found that feeding dietary calcium to those affected did little to improve bone density. This is because of certain hormonal changes that come along with aging. It was discovered that osteoporosis occurs because the person was never adequately mineralized earlier in life. She didn't get enough calcium as a youngster. As a result, she did not have enough calcium reserve in the bank and simply exhausted what precious little she did have in her reserve account. As hormonal levels change with menopause, bone deposition of calcium is more difficult and our reserves are drawn upon. This is why feeding calcium after the hormonal changes of menopause fails to result in increased bone density. To prevent nutritional diseases and a general breakdown of health, we must be careful to always have adequate minerals, vitamins, and enzymes in our food supply.

We must never forget that all the food we eat comes from the soil. The soil is the very base of the food chain. The soil is our greatest life-giver. Where the soil is poor, so is the health. It is tragic that some of the best soil in the world was right here in the United States and has been ruined by poor agricultural practices, poor soil management, and chemical farming. Although food is still grown in abundance, with the necessity of increasing the amounts of chemical fertilizers, it has suffered from poor quality, lacking in the all-important organic trace minerals. We are finally beginning to find out the truth: nature has no substitute.

Some years ago, the FDA mandated that the trace mineral iodine be added to table salt. The result is what we know as "iodized salt." Adding iodine was begun because of the recognition that our soils are depleted of this important trace mineral that is so necessary for the proper functioning of the thyroid gland. But, I'm wondering if the iodine added to salt is an organic, biochemical iodine or an inorganic, chemical iodine? Fortunately, of late, we have been returning to organic farming methods and restoring the soil's fertility. We are beginning to awaken to the fact that we can only be as healthy as our soil. My book *Empty Harvest*, co-authored with Mark Anderson, goes into detail concerning how our soils have become depleted and what the results have been. Artificial, laboratory-synthesized "foods" simply can neither build nor maintain health. These artificially contrived, chemical concoctions are what Adelle Davis called "foodless foods."

NUTRITION, THE MASTER SCIENCE

Nutrition is the master healing science. All else is mere remedy at best. Nutrition necessitates lifestyle change, while other methods, effective as they may seem, are temporary if nutritional changes are neglected. We cannot hope to get well by taking medication and consuming junk food. A spoonful of sugar may help the medicine go down, but it was too many spoonfuls of sugar that necessitated the medicine in the first place! It is my belief that all other therapeutic disciplines are secondary to nutrition.

I include in nutrition the care and feeding of the mind. This is mental and spiritual nutrition. Spiritual food came out of a land flowing with milk and honey (and the milk was raw goat's milk!). It is our nutrition that feeds our cells and causes tissue changes in our iris. Nutrition is the Master Science and stands above all other sciences in the healing arts. I believe that iris analysis is wedded to nutrition. I call them inseparable marriage partners, united for all time.

In Germany, as well as in some other European countries,

iris analysis is closely tied to homeopathic medicine. This is especially so in Germany because Germany is the birthplace of homeopathy. In Germany, in fact, iris analysis has been wedded more to homeopathic principles than to nutrition. Homeopathic medicines, unlike the more crude drugs of allopathy, are greatly refined. They contain none of the gross, inorganic, chemical preparations that are common in allopathic medicine. They, thus, do not produce any settlements that eventually discolor the iris. Homeopathic remedies affect the body at a higher, yet more subtle, vibrational level than do crude drugs. This is why they have no side effects. Homeopathic medicine is a great asset to the iridologist. It has long been respected in the field of natural therapeutics. When combined with the nutritional therapies, homeopathic medicine becomes an even more powerful tool to aid nature in restoring health.

Chiropractic is the second largest healing profession in the United States. It's literally growing by leaps and bounds, vaulting across continents to establish itself in many countries worldwide. Like homeopathy, it employs only natural therapeutics. Chiropractors use their hands to manually check and align the spinal column, thereby facilitating proper nerve flow to all tissues. It was the founder of this natural healing art, David Daniel Palmer, who remarked, "Disease is a condition caused by nerves being excited or depressed, deranging their functions." Since all nerves either emanate from, or terminate in, the brain, with the great majority entering or exiting from the various spinal levels, mechanical vertebral alignment that assures proper nerve flow is essential to better health. There is no other discipline that can perform painless techniques of spinal alignment to restore proper nerve flow as well as chiropractic. Chiropractic and iris analysis complement each other extremely well. In fact, an increasing number of iridologists are members of the chiropractic profession.

Herbology is yet another practice used by people who wish to abide by nature's ways. More than a few iridologists also practice herbal medicine. American Indian lore, as well as the traditions of Europe and the Far East, are rich in the historical use of herbs to restore and maintain health. In fact, even most uncivilized cultures have a long history of herbal use. (We should be careful whom we deem to be uncivilized!) We should also remember that many of our most effective allopathic medications were originally compounded from herbal extracts. In fact, many people who trained in medicine in the early years relied mainly on herbal preparations as their "medicine." Nowadays, many of the herbal essences used in allopathic medicine are isolated and synthetically reproduced in the laboratory, creating powerful but crude manhandled drugs. Herbs are still in popular use in many countries and, in some, constitute part of the orthodox health-care system. In China, for example, people can choose between traditional medicine (herbs and acupuncture) and Western medicine (drugs and surgery). The proper use of herbs to restore health is a valuable constituent of nature's pharmacy. More than a few practicing iridologists are also master herbalists. Herbs are food as well as medicine. "Let your medicine be your food," said Hippocrates.

Naturopathic physicians use a multitude of natural therapeutics—such as heliotherapy (sunlight), cryotherapy (cold), and hydrotherapy (water)—to effect curative changes in the body. They also employ the art and science of nutrition, herbs, manipulation, and exercise. The naturopaths and homeopaths were the ones who quickly embraced the concepts of iris analysis. To them goes the lion's share of the credit for the continued professional development of iris analysis. Doctors of naturopathy are common on the European continent and, at one time, were widely associated with health spas and sanitariums in the United States. As with homeopathy and other natural-health-care professions, however, subsequent legislation and medical politics all but eliminated the legal practice of naturopathy in the United States, a shameful and tragic loss of the freedom of choice in health care.

Allopathic physicians—doctors of medicine, as we know them—are trained to respond to illness with an arsenal of medicaments and drugs. They also practice surgery as a means of correction and an aid to healing. Many lives that otherwise would have been lost have been saved through allopathic practices. Iridology does not teach against the *proper* use of drugs or the employment of *necessary* and *expert* surgery. It recognizes that these responses are sometimes needed to save lives, make pain more bearable, and, in the case of surgery, to aid nature in the re-establishment of health. But through iridology, we frequently see how drugs and surgery are abused. We have become a society of drug abusers. Iridology and natural therapeutics try to keep us mindful that we should always consider drugs and surgery as emergency therapies or treatments to be employed only when more-natural therapies have failed. This is an idea whose time has come and is representative of prudent, conservative medicine. A growing number of medical physicians are coming around to feeling this way. This idea will someday lead us away from the abuse of drugs and surgery. It will draw us instead to a renewed appreciation that the healing power of nature is contained within food and the self, not in the synthesized nostrums of the pharmacy. It is the hope and desire of most iridologists—and, indeed of most alternative-health-care professionals—that allopathic medicine work in concert with them in the investigation and pursuit of health and healing. And, in fact, orthodox medicine has of late jumped on the nutrition bandwagon and is frantically trying to play catch-up ball in teaching nutrition to medical students after years of discounting its role in maintaining health.

There are many schools of healing based upon nature's principles. My purpose is not to list them all, but to acquaint you with the idea that any therapy that works in accordance with nature may prove beneficial. All have their therapeutic niche. The *Heilpraktor* (health practitioner) in Germany uses iridology in his natural therapeutic work. In fact, there are more than 3,000 of these doctors in Germany. All natural-healing methods share a kinship with iris analysis.

It is wise to always be cautious in passing judgment on another healing art. Those who are not cautious usually pass judgment out of ignorance. Man has much to learn about the plant Earth, the physical body that his life force animates, and the unseen-yet-real forces that govern his existence and well-being. It behooves each of us to consider favorably and honorably all those who act in a spirit of good will, with purity of heart, in their endeavor to provide health care. In all our efforts to regain and sustain health, we must be careful never to engage in any practice that might bring harm to a person. "First do no harm" is the ancient and initial commandment of all true healing. It is through iris analysis that we can observe a return to health, a restoration of tissue integrity, with the employment of nutrition. *No therapeutic regimen without the complement of nutrition will cause healing lines to appear in the iris.*

The science of iridology should no longer be overlooked. Neither should it be winked at by those who look condescendingly upon things they do not understand. Iridology needs to be taken seriously, the same way that nutrition, of late, has begun to be given the consideration it so rightfully deserves. There is no reason to further delay research in iridology. The pioneers who gave their time, talent, and energy in the development and clinical practice of iridology and nutrition can no longer be ignored.

THE LEGAL PRACTICE OF IRIS ANALYSIS

Despite much progress in iris analysis, its practice is not presently licensed in any of the fifty states. Therefore, in no state is an iris-analysis practitioner allowed by law to either diagnose or treat disease. As we have learned, however, due to a different understanding of health, iridology is not associated with diagnosing or treating disease.

Barring the legal prohibition or regulation of practicing iris analysis in a particular state, a person is usually free to engage in providing this service *providing he does not diagnose or treat disease.* However, always check the laws of your particular state.

At the present time, there is no accredited curriculum that is universally used to teach iris analysis. There are no duly required examinations for iridologists, although many who teach iridology do require their students to pass comprehensive examinations to qualify for a certificate of course completion.

For duly licensed health-care providers, it is usually against state law to claim skills (such as iris analysis) that might appear to set them apart from their peers. For instance, a person cannot be a licensed chiropractor and, on his chiropractic sign or advertisement, state also that he is an iridologist since iris analysis is not a customary and recognized part of chiropractic practice. In so doing, the chiropractor would be appearing to set himself apart from other members of his profession. Again, it is prudent to check your state laws regarding the practice of iris analysis even if you are a licensed health professional.

IRIDOLOGY EDUCATION

Responsible iridologists are perhaps harsher critics than anyone else of what they do. They are the first to point out the limitations of iris analysis as well as the benefits. More than anyone, they have firsthand knowledge of research begging to be conducted in the effort to provide concrete answers to the tough questions in iridology. Every iridologist would likely admit that the sum total of his knowledge is far less than the answers he seeks.

Those who use iris analysis know that it works. They know that it proves itself clinically—in practice—where results count. Who can argue with success? After all, iris analysis as a practiced technique is successful. It has a long history and it works.

Until recently, all iridologists were either self-taught from correspondence courses prepared by practicing iridologists or from textbooks and other literature on the subject. A few were directly tutored by a master iridologist. What many lacked in credentials, they made up for in enthusiasm and dedication.

More than a few iridologists came from among the ranks of the long-recognized drugless healing professions, both here and abroad. These people possessed professional degrees, had clinical experience in health care, and not infrequently were graduates of respected schools. A few were doctors of medicine, as was Ignatz von Peczely, the founder of iris analysis.

Education in iris analysis can today be obtained through correspondence courses, through the private study of iridology textbooks, and by attending courses given in various cities in the United States, Canada, Latin America, Australia, and Europe. Recently, Hawaii became the home of the first recognized institution to offer earned degrees in herbology, acupuncture, and iridology. The College of Oriental Medicine is part of the University of Health Sciences, in Honolulu.

For a list of addresses and phone numbers for obtaining information on iridology courses and educational materials, please see "For More Information," on page 157.

COMPUTERIZED IRIS ANALYSIS

The present time is being characterized as the "data age," the age of information processing. Why shouldn't iridology be a part of it? I believe it should. Currently under development through Bernard Jensen International, Inc., is the Neuroptic Scanning Computer. Iridology has been waiting a long time for the computer to arrive. With the computer, we can digitize the image of an iris from a color video camera and feed the digitized image directly into the computer. Then, the computer can analyze the image using a database developed by skilled iridologists who have been working closely with professional computer programmers. My sixty-two years of clinical iridology and nutritional experience, combined with the many years of practice of my associates, are helping to create a major advancement in the field of computerized iris analysis.

The computerization of iris analysis will assure objectivity in the examination process from iris to iris and from person to person. The iris analyses of a single subject at different times can be accurately compared. And, iris changes too minute to be seen with a magnifier, to say nothing of the naked eye, will be seen by the computer and recorded. This special ability of the computer to see in finer detail and with greater accuracy than is possible by the naked eye will bring out many heretofore undreamed-of possibilities in both the scope and accuracy of iris analysis. Many possibilities are associated with the employment of digital electronic analysis of the iris. You, the reader, can use your imagination. All will come in time.

Computers, however, will likely be a mixed blessing. I have said in my lectures many times that we can have whatever we want in life, but we must take what comes with it. In the same vein, Theodore Parker Ferris, the famous preacher and rector of Trinity Church in Boston, once preached a sermon entitled, "The Blight Behind the Blessing." He said that we can't have something new and wonderful without the troubles that come along with it. There are going to be some other new things coming along with the new computer technology. Computerized iris analysis is no doubt going to point up new areas that will need to be incorporated into the iris chart. And, I think, it will show us where we have been making some errors. Some of our preconceived notions will no doubt be altered. The iris chart will change as thousands of irides are subjected to the computer's digital scrutiny. All these changes, of course, will serve to create an iris chart with much greater accuracy. That is part of the blessing. We must be prepared to accept and incorporate the changes.

I'm sure that the most exciting new information will concern the brain areas. I expect this new information to greatly enlighten our understanding of the mental side of health and well-being. I also expect the statistical compilations of the thousands of computer-analyzed irides to finally prove true certain key concepts long held by iridologists. For one, I certainly expect the computer to confirm the relationship of the digestive tract to every organ and function in the body. Once accepted and taught outside of iridology, this concept alone will bring improved health to millions.

Also being explored currently by Bernard Jensen International are various other cutting edge technologies that bode well for the science of iridology. I foresee an iridologist in clinical practice being able to send digital images of an iris directly to a distant computer over the telephone lines. The computer will analyze the iris and return the results within minutes, printing them out in the iridologist's office. The technology to do this is here now. Many new things will be possible in the future because of the digital-based information age.

IRIDOLOGY RESEARCH

We cannot deny that iris analysis begs for proper scientific protocol followed by unbiased research. Some people claim that this has already been accomplished and that the question of the validity of iris analysis has been laid to rest. In recent years, some people have attempted to disprove the claims made by the practitioners of iris analysis. They say that the so-called research was badly flawed because proper protocols were never established. What iridology needs is to obtain the services of unbiased, competent researchers to establish proper protocols for continued iridological research. The next step should then be for the research to be carried out with integrity by qualified individuals, according to the newly established protocols. Truth will prevail.

It's up to you now. You are the one who must collect your thoughts and make a decision about the value of iridology. You are the one who must observe, test, experiment, and record. You are the one who must decide to let it drop or pursue more advanced knowledge of the subject. Please remember that iridology is a grassroots science. It has come to where it is through the interest of people just like you. It is well to re-member that most good and valuable ideas rise up from the bottom. The trickle-down theory works well for water, but grav-itational force has no effect on the leaven of ideas. They rise. If iridology is to blossom and flourish, it cannot be left to the labor of scholars in the halls of medical academia. Even the experts admit that battles are won by the troops in the field. There is something to be said for being a good soldier.

A good soldier, however, is not a "true believer." Iridology is not a cult. It is not an ideological movement. It requires nothing of its adherents but good faith, an open mind, and searching for the truth. Like the tissue condition it hopes to reveal, it expects nothing more from the student than good integrity. Reading this book does not qualify anyone as an "iridologist." My sin-cere hope is that the reader realizes that this book only scratches the surface of what is an extensive and even lifelong pursuit. I have lived with iridology as a friend for over sixty-two years and still feel like a child, amazed equally at what I have learned and what I have yet to discover. The secrets iridology still holds drive me onward, with that which has been revealed serving as my sustenance. Iridology has been waiting for you for a long time. Where have you been?

Appendices

Appendix A

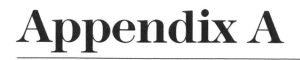

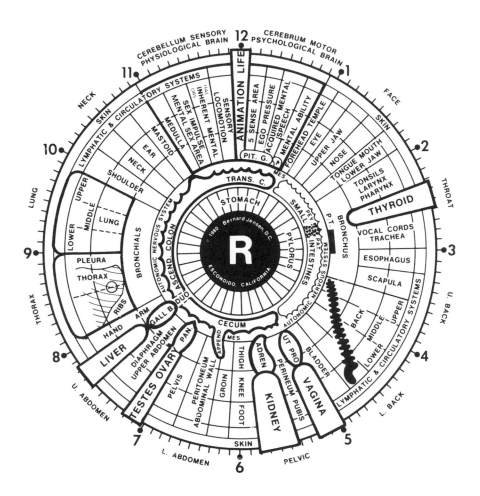

RIGHT IRIS
P — Pineal
Pey Pat — Peyers Patches
Mes — Mesentery
Hal — Hallucination
P.T. — Parathyroid

Jensen Chart

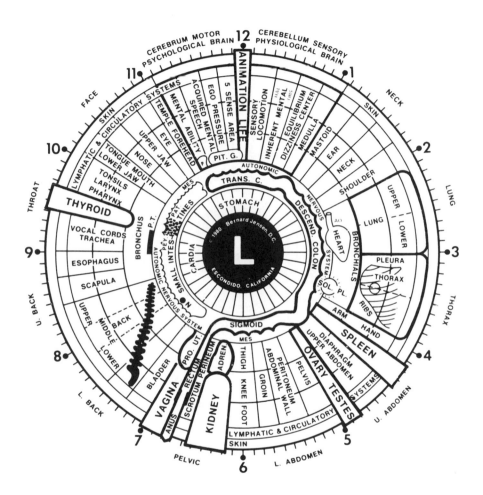

LEFT IRIS
Pit. G. — Pituitary Gland
Sol. Pl. — Solar Plexus
N — Navel
Obs — Obsession
AO — Aorta

Appendix B

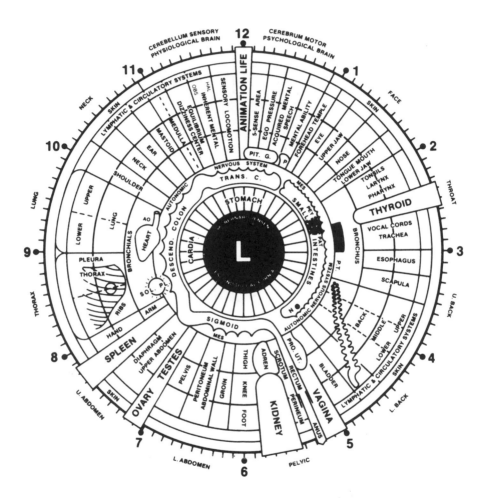

LEFT IRIS
Pit. G. — Pituitary Gland
Sol. Pl. — Solar Plexus
N — Navel
Obs — Obsession
AO — Aorta

Reverse Jensen Chart

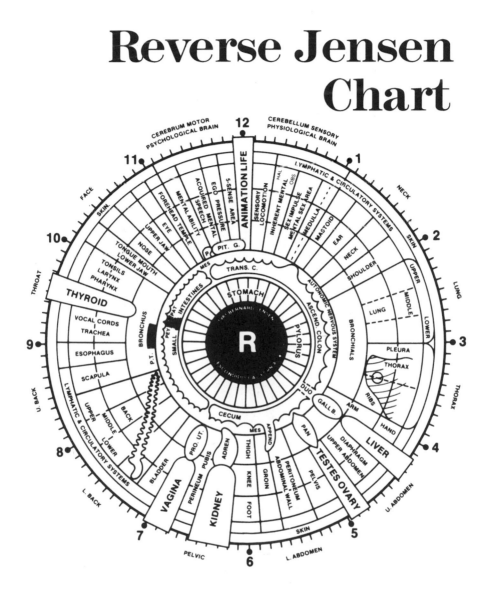

RIGHT IRIS
P — Pineal
Pey Pat — Peyers Patches
Mes — Mesentery
Hal — Hallucination
P.T. — Parathyroid

Appendix C
Iris Signs

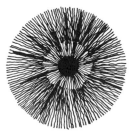

Radii solaris

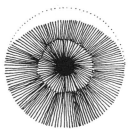

Arcus senilis

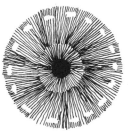

Lymphatic rosary

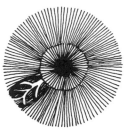

Healing lines

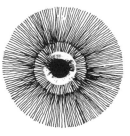

Overactive stomach

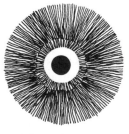

Underactive stomach

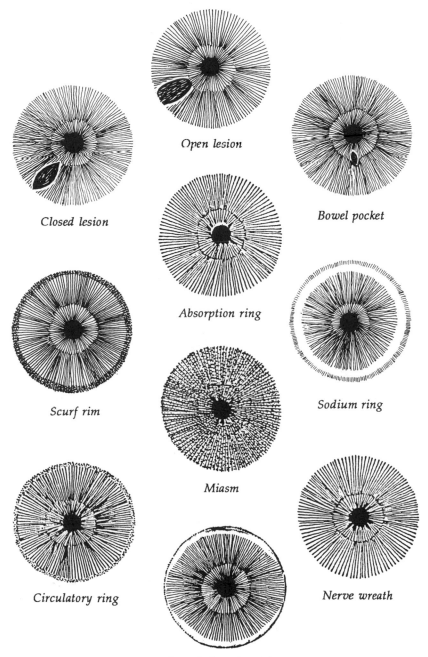

Open lesion

Closed lesion

Bowel pocket

Absorption ring

Scurf rim

Sodium ring

Miasm

Circulatory ring

Nerve wreath

Anemia in extremities

Appendix D
New Discoveries

Visions of Health is all about the still evolving art and science of iridology. As so often happens with a subject in that stage of development, fresh discoveries are constantly being made. It has happened here. After this book was typeset, brand new findings were announced by Bernard Jensen International researchers concerning the utilization of the modern computer in iris analysis.

NEW DEVELOPMENTS IN COMPUTERIZED IRIS ANALYSIS

The research being conducted of late at Bernard Jensen International has concentrated on how to use the computer to aid in our understanding of what can be revealed in the iris. Since the surface of the iris can, with the aid of the computer, be viewed as the three-dimensional topographic map that it truly is, the newer computer technologies can provide the iridology researcher with enhanced and detailed graphics of actual iris topography. Alterations in the topography reflect not only inherent, genetic patterns but also modifications in these patterns brought about by diet, environment, and lifestyle. By assigning colors to the computer gray-scale image, vivid examples of iris topography can be achieved. In addition, using a grid that looks like a net draped over the topography of the iris aids greatly in enhancing depth of field.

Because the elevations and depressions above and below a "normal" baseline represent the activity, or energy, of iris fibers, acute through degenerative states can be graphically depicted.

"Normal" is construed as a fine line between acute and sub-acute. When fibers are acute, they are more active than normal and in an excess-energy state. This causes them to appear raised above the "normal" on the iris topographical map, the same way that an elevated area such as a mountain appears raised above the average terrain.

As iris fibers become subacute, they become less active and descend to a lower-than-normal energy state, appearing depressed on the iris topographical map. As an area becomes chronic and its iris fibers sink to yet lower energy states, the fibers form hollows in the iris surface. Degenerative states severely lack energy and form the bottom of the deepest depressions. Degenerative states are evidenced on gray-scale illustrations (see Figures A.1 and A.2 on page 156) as very dark gray tones, almost black.

On Figure A.1, note the active, elevated section representing the autonomic nerve wreath, as well as the depression representing a chronic condition and inherent weakness in the heart area. In Figure A.2, observe again the raised, active fibers representing the nerve wreath and also the depression indicating underactive, low-energy fibers representing the degenerative state of a bowel pocket. The pocket is located just inside the autonomic nerve wreath in the area of the descending colon.

Pay particular attention to how the autonomic nerve wreath splits into two branches in Figure A.2 to form the chronic depression lesion associated with a classic heart weakness. Also notice the section of a small healing line forming in the center of the heart lesion, indicated by the raised plateau. This latter is referred to as a "healing line" in iridology because fibers within the depression are beginning to raise up with renewed energy and activity, creating the appearance of a butte or mesa within the greater depression. This regaining of energy and raising of the iris fibers is a reversal of direction from the chronic downhill progression and is consistent with Hering's law. We must go through this reversal process in order to achieve true healing and be on the road to recovery.

These findings are just the tip of the iceberg. As computers become more refined, and their programmers and users more adept, new research developments concerning iris analysis will pour in. This appendix will become a book of its own.

Figure A.1

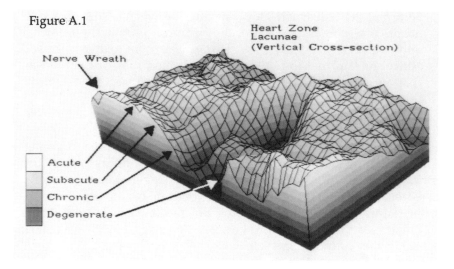

These computer-generated gray-scales depict cross-sections of a heart zone. Figure A.1 shows a vertical cross-section; Figure A.2 shows a horizontal cross-section.

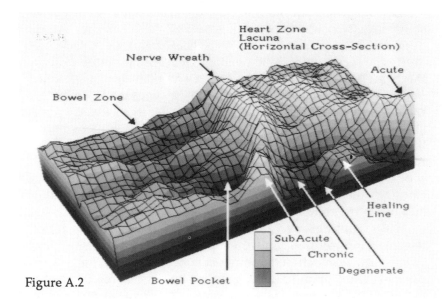

Figure A.2

For More Information

For more information on anything discussed in this book, plus information on iridology courses, educational seminars, and lectures by Dr. Jensen, please write to the authors at the following addresses:

Dr. Bernard Jensen
Bernard Jensen International, Inc.
24360 Old Wagon Road
Escondido, CA 92027

Dr. Donald V. Bodeen
Bernard Jensen International, Inc.
219 New Hackensack Road
Poughkeepsie, NY 12603

Dr. Jensen is also the founder and president of Iridologists International, an international association of iridologists that is devoted to iridology research and advancement. Membership includes subscriptions to the quarterly journals *Iris Wisdom and the Allied Healing Arts* and *In Search of Excellence: A Newer Concept of Nutrition.* For more information on the organization and its work, write to:

Iridologists International
24360 Old Wagon Road
Escondido, CA 92027

The use of the computer in iris analysis will be discussed in detail in upcoming issues of *Iris Wisdom and the Allied Healing Arts*. For subscription information, please write to Iridologists International at the address on page 157.

For more information on the courses and degrees offered by the College of Oriental Medicine, please write to:

> College of Oriental Medicine
> University of Health Sciences
> Graduate Division
> 181 South Kukui Street
> Suite 206
> Honolulu, HI 96813

To reach Dr. Willie Hauser or the Pastor Felke Institute, please write to:

> Pastor Felke Institute
> Heidestr. 3
> 7258 Heimsheim
> Germany

Glossary

Allopathic. Used to describe those health-care practices that employ drugs for the treatment of disease. Medical doctors are allopathic physicians.

Amorphous. An adjective describing a shape not well-defined. In iridology, it describes a special type of grid that is laid over photos of irides to help in the analysis of those irides. It departs from the more stylized types of grids and more closely resembles the actual shape of the iris. In particular, its intestinal areas reflect an alteration in shape to more closely conform with actual observations.

Anemia. A medical term indicating a lack of adequate blood flow to an area. An anemic condition of the body in general may result when the blood is not properly constituted.

Arcus senilis. A gray to milky crescent-shaped settlement covering the uppermost portion of the iris. For the iridologist, it indicates brain anemia.

Arrhythmia. A disruption of normal, regular rhythm. In medicine, it usually pertains to the heartbeat.

Autonomic nerve wreath. Sometimes called the "nerve wreath," "iris frill," or, simply, "the wreath." It is the raised, irregular iris landmark encircling the pupil, usually located about one-third of the distance from the pupil circumference to the iris boundary. It is unique to every individual, just like fingerprints. In iridology, it represents the autonomic nervous system.

Candida albicans. A yeast organism that can become pathogenic if left uncontrolled. It is usually a problem only in people with compromised tissue integrity, depressed immunity, or imbalances often associated with heavy or prolonged antibiotic use.

Cornea. The normally transparent, dome-like cover over the iris.

Discrete fiber. A single, distinct iris fiber. In great numbers, it makes up the stroma, or structure, of the iris. Each discrete fiber is actually composed of many microscopic-sized fiber bundles.

Erythrocyte sedimentation rate (ESR). The measured rate at which red blood cells settle out of blood serum when the blood serum is left standing, undisturbed, in a test tube for a predetermined length of time. A higher rate than normal suggests an inflammatory response in the body. The higher the rate, the more extensive the inflammation.

Fiberoptic. An optical or light-transmitting device that employs multiple strands of flexible glass or plastic to transmit light. One of its advantages is that it transmits light around corners and over lengthy distances with minimal loss. Another advantage, especially for iridology, is that the transmitted light is cold since it is removed from its heat source, thereby also reducing the danger of lamp explosion.

Flexure. A bend. The flexures of the colon are the points at which the colon alters its course by bending more than 90 degrees. The splenic flexure is near the spleen.

Homeostasis. The condition of the body when all its cells are working in balance, resulting in a state of perfect well-being.

Irides. Plural of "iris."

Kinesiology. The study of muscle function and action; of body movement and its resultant effects.

Miasm. An adulteration or pollution. In iridology, a miasmic iris is sometimes called a "dishwater eye" because it resembles dirty dishwater in color. It has had its normal color brilliance altered by years of wrong living habits and sometimes from exposure to drugs, pollutants, or chemicals. It looks dull, dirty, and off-color.

Nostrums. Drugs and medicaments used to suppress diseases and symptoms, and usually purchased over-the-counter.

Ophthalmology. The branch of medicine concerned with diseases of the eye and their treatment.

Parasympathetic. One of the major classifications of nervous-system tissue in the body. It is the nervous system that serves functionally as a counterbalance to the sympathetic nervous system.

Pathogen. An entity such as a bacteria, virus, yeast, etc., that can be associated with a disease state. Unlike orthodox medical practitioners, adherents to natural medicine do not consider these traditional pathogens to be the cause of disease but merely associated with certain diseases.

Pleura. The membrane lining the chest cavity. The inflammation of this membrane is known as "pleurisy."

Pupillary ruff. Another name for the assimilation ring. It is a rough or serrated brown or reddish-brown area that is evidenced, if present, immediately inside the pupil circumference.

Radii solaris. Literally, "rays of the sun." In iridology, this is an inherent weakness that resembles, in appearance, bicycle spokes extending out from near the autonomic nerve wreath or close to the pupil. When there are several spokes, they look like rays of the sun, with the pupil the sun.

Reflexology. The broad spectrum of sciences, including iridology, based upon the neurological fact that all the parts of the body are linked to, and affected by the stimulation of, certain other parts through the central nervous system.

Silicosis. An acquired lung condition caused by repeated exposure to abnormal amounts of silicon dust. In the past, this was an industrial hazard in some jobs. It causes a thick mucous secretion, cough, pain, and, eventually, respiratory dysfunction.

Sphincter. A circular muscle surrounding a natural opening that serves to control the size of that opening. The pupil is an example of an opening controlled by a sphincter muscle.

Tissue integrity. The inherent strength or construction of a tissue. The soundness of a tissue.

Topography. The detailed description of the surface features of an area. In iridology, it refers to the surface features of the iris.

Vascular. Pertaining to the blood vessels of the body.

Wholistic. Describes something that takes the whole person into consideration, as opposed to just certain segments, when used in connection with health care. Wholism is the concept that a person is more than the sum of his discrete biological parts.

Zones. In iridology, the areas defined on the iris chart by concentric circles, with the pupil as the center. Iris charts usually have seven zones.

Bibliography

Davidson, Victor S. *Iridiagnosis.* Wellingborough, England: Thorsons Publishers Ltd., 1979.

Deck, Josef. *Differentiation of Iris Markings.* Translated by R. Freystuck-Baynham, Ulrike Fuchs, and Hans-Jurgen Fuchs. 2d ed. Ettlingen, Germany: J. Deck, 1982.

———. *Principles of Iris Diagnosis.* Translated by R. Freystuck-Baynham, Ulrike Fuchs, and Hans-Jurgen Fuchs. Ettlingen, Germany: J. Deck, 1982.

Hall, Dorothy. *Iridology: How the Eyes Reveal Your Health and Your Personality.* New Canaan, Conn.: Keats Publishing, Inc. 1980.

Jenks, Jim. *The Eyes Have It: An Introduction to Iridology.* Provo, Utah: Bi World, 1978.

Jensen, Bernard. *Beyond Basic Health.* Garden City Park, N.Y.: Avery Publishing Group, 1988.

———. *Iridology: The Science and Practice in the Healing Arts, Volume II.* Escondido, Calif.: Bernard Jensen, 1982.

———. *Iridology Simplified.* Escondido, Calif.: Bernard Jensen, 1980.

———. *The Science and Practice of Iridology.* Escondido, Calif.: Bernard Jensen, 1952.

Jensen, B., and Sylvia Bell. *Tissue Cleansing Through Bowel Management.* Escondido, Calif.: Bernard Jensen, 1981.

Kriege, Theodor. *Fundamental Basis of Irisdiagnosis.* Translated by A. W. Priest. Essex, England: L. N. Fowler & Co., Ltd., 1969.

Kritzer, J. Haskel. *Text-Book of Iridiagnosis.* Chicago: J. H. Kritzer, 1924.

Lahn, Edward Henry. *Iridology, the Diagnosis From the Eye.* Evanston, Ill.: Kosmos Publishing Co., 1914.

Liljequist, Niels. *Diagnosis From the Eye.* Rockford, Ill.: Iridology Publishing Co., 1916.

Lindlahr, Henry. *Natural Therapeutics: Iridiagnosis and Other Diagnostic Methods.* Chicago: Lindlahr Publishing Co., 1919.

Schneider, Glenda. *Iris Analysis: A Practical Guide to Revealing Amazing Secrets Through the Iris.* Santee, Calif.: W & G Publishing, 1982.

Vriend, John. *Eyes Talk: Through Iridology to Better Health.* Melbourne, Australia: Lothian Publishing Co. Pty Ltd., 1988.

Wilborn, R., J. Terrell, and M. Terrell. *Handbook of Iridiagnosis and Rational Therapy.* Mokelumne Hill, Calif.: Health Research, 1961.

About the Authors

Dr. Bernard Jensen

One of America's foremost pioneering nutritionists, Dr. Bernard Jensen began his career in 1929 as a chiropractic physician. He soon turned to the art of nutrition in search of remedies for his own health problems. In his formative years, Dr. Jensen studied under such giants as Dr. Benedict Lust, Dr. John Tilden, Dr. John H. Kellogg, and Dr. V. G. Rocine. Later, he observed first-hand the cultural practices of people in more than fifty-five countries, discovering important links between food and health.

Dr. Jensen has also taught around the world, including in some of the more exotic cities of the Orient. He was invited by the Chinese government to teach iridology on mainland China and by the Taiwanese to set up a Department of Iridology at a large veterans' hospital in Taipai. He also spent twenty-seven days teaching iridology classes in Malaysia to enthusiastic students. In 1955, Dr. Jensen established the Hidden Valley Ranch in Escondido, California, as a retreat and learning center dedicated to the healing principles of nature.

Over the years, Dr. Jensen has received a multitude of prestigious awards and honors for his work in nutrition and the healing arts. These honors include Knighthood in the Order of

St. John of Malta, the Dag Hammarskjold Peace Award of Belgium, and an award from Queen Juliana of the Netherlands. He is also the author of numerous articles and best-selling books. At age eighty-three, he continues to teach, travel, and learn.

Dr. Donald Bodeen

Dr. Donald Bodeen is a chiropractor in private practice in his hometown of Poughkeepsie, New York. He began his career in 1976 after receiving his doctorate in chiropractic from the National College of Chiropractic at Lombard, Illinois. He also holds the degree of Doctor of Iridology, which he received from the College of Oriental Medicine, University of Health Sciences; a bachelor degree in human biology; and a bachelor degree in aviation technology. In addition, he is an ordained minister. It was while serving in this last capacity that he became interested in healing, his own health having been compromised. Today, as a health practitioner, he feels that people are a unique blend of the physical, mental, and spiritual, and he treats them as such. He feels that "we have hopes, fears, joys, and loves all blended to create varying lifestyles and outlooks, making each person the unique creature that he is."

Along with his many years of learning, Dr. Bodeen has also spent many years teaching. He has lectured to various groups in the Dutchess County (New York) area and around the country. He has taught classes at the State University of New York at New Paltz and has lectured at Marist College in Poughkeepsie. He has been a guest on several radio talk shows.

Iridology, in particular, is close to Dr. Bodeen's heart. He is a long-time student of Dr. Jensen, with whom he has become close friends. He is a contributor to the world's foremost textbook on iridology, *Iridology: The Science and Practice in the Healing Arts, Volume II*, authored by Dr. Jensen, and is a member of Iridologists International. He routinely takes iris photos of all his new chiropractic patients, using the latest available technology in iris cameras.

Away from work, Dr. Bodeen enjoys amateur "ham" radio, hiking, photography, and travel. He and his wife, Joyce, have two sons.

Index

If You've Enjoyed Reading This Book . . .

. . . why not tell a friend about it? If you're interested in learning more about Dr. Bernard Jensen's approach to health, here are some other titles you may find to be informative, engaging, and fun.

Vibrant Health From Your Kitchen

A warm and wonderful tour through Dr. Jensen's latest discoveries about food, nutrition, and health, this book provides the guidance needed to keep your family disease-free, healthy, and happy.

Tissue Cleansing Through Bowel Management

Toxin-laden tissue can become a breeding ground for disease. This remarkable book instructs you in the removal of toxins and the restoration of health and youthfulness through the cleansing and care of the organs of elimination.

Food Healing for Man

We now know that foods can repair the tissue damage that accompanies most illness and disease. Look over the shoulders of the great pioneer nutritionists as they investigate the links between nutrition and disease.

Chlorella: Gem of the Orient

Why does Dr. Jensen consider chlorella—a green alga—the most valuable broad-spectrum food supplement discovery of the twentieth century? You'll find out in this unusually beautiful, fully illustrated, hard cover book.

Nature Has a Remedy

This popular classic provides a delightful description of the many paths to natural healing—foods, herbs, exercise, climate selection, personology, and hundreds of effective remedies.

World Keys to Health and Long Life

Based on Dr. Jensen's travels to over fifty-five countries, this fascinating book describes the health and longevity secrets of centenarians interviewed in the Hunza Valley of India; Vilcabamba, Peru; the Caucasus Mountains of the Soviet Union; and other places around the world.

Doctor-Patient Handbook

Discover the reversal process and healing crisis that Nature uses to rid the body of disease and restore well-being. Here is a fresh approach to wholistic health.

Dr. Jensen's Real Soup & Salad Book

Enjoy a delicious collection of time-tested recipes that nourish and heal the body while satisfying the soul.

Slender Me Naturally

Dr. Jensen's answer to fad diets that don't work is a natural weight loss program that does. Developed over fifty-eight years of experience with overweight patients, this program is a healthful and effective way of losing unwanted weight.

Breathe Again Naturally

Get rid of asthma, allergies, bronchitis, hay fever, and other respiratory problems. Dr. Jensen discusses nutrition, herbs that work, food supplements, breathing exercises, attitude, and climate.

Arthritis, Rheumatism and Osteoporosis

Are you among the one in four Americans who suffers from arthritis, rheumatism, or osteoporosis? Would you like to know what to do about it? This book is for you.

Foods That Heal

This book presents the basic principles of Hippocrates, Dr. Rocine, and Dr. Jensen regarding the use of foods to help the body regain health. The author has also included a complete guide to the various fruits and vegetables we all need.

In Search of Shangri-La

Here is the very personal journal of Dr. Jensen's physical and spiritual travels through China into Tibet, and his reflections on his search for Shangri-La.

Beyond Basic Health

Dr. Jensen looks at the deteriorating state of modern man's health and offers practical advice˙and insights to those health professionals who must deal with today's devastating illnesses.

Love, Sex and Nutrition

Based on years of detailed study, this book explores the link between diet, sensuality, and relationships. This is an important and practical guide for people who wish to improve their sexuality safely and naturally.

Empty Harvest

This book explains the relationship between soil and man—how when we pollute and rape the soil, we destroy our own immune systems. It also offers suggestions on how we can detoxify and cleanse both ourselves and the Earth.

For information regarding prices, write to:

Bernard Jensen International   Tel.: (619) 749-2727
24360 Old Wagon Road   Fax: (619) 749-1248
Escondido, California 92027-9667